# CONTENTS

Free eBook: Digital Detox to Unplug & Heal: Navigating a World Without Screens — 3

Chapter 1: Introduction to Intermittent Fasting — 6

Chapter 2: Evolutionary Basis for Fasting — 15

Chapter 3: The Female Physiology & Fasting — 24

Chapter 4: Common Fasting Protocols — 33

Chapter 5: Fasting and Weight Loss for Women — 42

Chapter 6: Fasting and Muscle Maintenance — 52

Chapter 7: Mental and Cognitive Benefits — 61

Chapter 8: Aging, Longevity, and Fasting — 71

Chapter 9: Fasting and Hormonal Balance — 81

Chapter 10: Fasting During Different Life Phases — 91

Chapter 11: Social and Lifestyle Aspects — 101

Chapter 12: Fasting and Gut Health — 111

Chapter 13: Potential Side Effects and Solutions — 121

Chapter 14: Integrating Nutrition with Fasting — 132

Chapter 15: Emotional and Psychological Aspects — 144

Chapter 16: Troubleshooting and Adjusting Protocols — 154

Chapter 17: Combining Fasting with Other Diets — 164

Chapter 18: Real-Life Testimonies — 174

Chapter 19: Tips for Long-term Success — 183

# Chapter 20: Concluding Thoughts

# Intermittent Fasting for Women of Any Age

## The Woman's Guide to Timeless Health and Wellness

Cypress Kingsley & Brighton Callaway

# FREE EBOOK: DIGITAL DETOX TO UNPLUG & HEAL: NAVIGATING A WORLD WITHOUT SCREENS

Want a free eBook teaching you how to do a digital detox and heal your brain from device addiction?

Visit our website to grab a free copy today!

www.selfhelp.academy

**Disclaimer**

We are so excited that you've picked up this book on intermittent fasting. Our goal is to share information, ideas, and experiences that might be of interest to you on your journey. We really hope you find this resource helpful and insightful.

Now, it's super important to mention that while this book is packed with information and research, it's not intended to replace professional medical, health, legal, or financial advice. We're not doctors or certified financial advisors, and this isn't a one-size-fits-all kind of deal.

Everyone's body and circumstances are unique, and it's essential to consult with a healthcare provider or a qualified professional for advice tailored to your individual needs, especially before making any significant changes to your diet, lifestyle, or financial situation.

We've done our best to ensure the accuracy and completeness of the information in this book, but we can't cover all possible situations or individual needs. Therefore, the author and publisher expressly disclaim responsibility for any adverse effects arising from the use or application of the information contained herein.

Please remember, the insights and perspectives shared in this book are based on the author's experiences, opinions, and research, and they may not necessarily align with your individual health needs or financial circumstances. So, while we hope you enjoy the read and gain some nuggets of wisdom, please use this book as a general guide and not as the ultimate source of legal, financial, or health advice.

Remember, the journey to health and well-being is a personal one, and it's important to be informed and make choices that are right for you. We wish you all the best on your journey and hope this book serves as a valuable companion along the way. Happy reading!

# CHAPTER 1: INTRODUCTION TO INTERMITTENT FASTING

## Part I: The Science Behind Fasting

Welcome! Let me begin by congratulating you on taking this transformative journey. Seeking knowledge is the first step towards making lasting changes in our lives. But why fasting? Let's delve deep, hand-in-hand, into the captivating world of fasting science to uncover the answers.

**The Beauty of Body Rhythms**

Our bodies are designed, or should I say, fine-tuned like a symphony orchestra. Just as a conductor ensures each instrument plays at the right time, our body has natural rhythms – our sleep-wake cycle, hunger pangs, and even that afternoon energy slump. Have you ever wondered about the magic that governs these patterns?

At the heart of this magic is our circadian rhythm – our internal body clock that regulates our 24-hour cycle. Interestingly, our digestive system, metabolism, and even cell repair processes follow this rhythm. Now, think about it: If we're constantly eating, when does our body find the time to rest, repair, and rejuvenate?

This is where intermittent fasting gracefully waltzes in.

## The Actual 'Break' in Breakfast

Remember the joy of waking up to the smell of breakfast? The term 'breakfast' is a direct nod to its purpose - to 'break the fast'. Historically, humans weren't habitual snackers. We didn't always have the luxury to pop open a fridge whenever we felt like it. Instead, our ancestors had periods of feast and famine. This is how our bodies, over time, adapted to efficiently using and storing energy.

When we eat, our body's immediate response is to turn the food into glucose (a type of sugar), providing us with immediate energy. What isn't used is stored in the liver as glycogen. Now, if our body runs out of this glucose? Ah, this is where the wonder begins! Our body starts converting stored fat into molecules called ketones, an alternative source of energy. This state is known as ketosis. And guess what? This natural process gets a boost during fasting.

## The Cellular Tidy-up

There's another absolutely fascinating thing that our body does when it's not busy digesting. It tidies up! Imagine your cells as rooms that have been used for a wild party. Over time, they gather waste and damaged parts. Enter autophagy (from the Greek 'auto', meaning 'self', and 'phagein', meaning 'eat'). During fasting, our cells start this self-cleaning process, where they remove the damaged bits, making way for regeneration. It's like spring cleaning for our cells, and oh, how they love it!

## The Hormonal Symphony

If there's one thing women are intimately familiar with, it's hormones. These incredible molecules dictate so much of our life, from our monthly cycles to our moods. When we talk about fasting, insulin is the superstar hormone. Every time we eat, our blood sugar rises, leading to insulin being released. Its job? To help our cells absorb this sugar. But here's the catch – with constant eating, our cells can become resistant to insulin's effects, leading to a cascade of health issues.

Fasting gives our body a break, allowing insulin levels to drop and cells to become more responsive. Essentially, it's like hitting the reset button on our metabolism.

**Harnessing the Benefits**

Now, with all this knowledge, it's essential to remember – every woman is unique. What works wonders for one might not for another. That's why understanding the science behind fasting is the cornerstone for tailoring it to our needs. And darling reader, we're just scratching the surface. The chapters ahead will dive deeper into the specific challenges and rewards women can encounter in the world of intermittent fasting.

But for now, just take a moment to marvel at the intricate dance our body performs, from cellular repair to metabolic balance. All we need to do is give it the time and space to do its job.

There you go! A deep dive into the beautiful, mesmerizing world of fasting science. Stay with me, and together, we'll unlock the countless secrets that can pave the way for a healthier, happier you.

# Chapter 1: Introduction to Intermittent Fasting
## Part II: Myths and Misconceptions

You know, every great journey - be it of self-discovery, health, or adventure - has its fair share of myths. These can sometimes be charming stories handed down through generations, but other times, they act as roadblocks, making us second guess our choices. Intermittent fasting, despite its deep roots and the science backing it up, is not exempt from these tales. So, let's don our detective hats and dispel some myths together, shall we?

### Myth 1: Fasting is just another diet fad

How many times have you heard this one? Oh, fasting, isn't that just another one of those trends? Now, here's the truth bomb: intermittent fasting isn't a "diet" in the conventional sense. It's not about what you eat, but when you eat. And it's certainly not new. Our ancestors practiced fasting out of necessity (think: hunters and gatherers waiting for their next meal). Many cultures also integrate fasting into spiritual practices. So, darling, it's not a fleeting trend – it's a time-tested lifestyle.

### Myth 2: Fasting leads to nutrient deficiency

A common concern is that fasting can deprive us of essential nutrients. In reality, fasting teaches us to be more mindful of what we consume during our eating windows. It's an opportunity to ensure we're packing in nutrient-dense foods, leading to a richer, more wholesome diet. Remember, it's about quality, not always quantity.

### Myth 3: It's starving yourself

Whoa, hold on a minute! Fasting is NOT about starving. Starvation is a severe and involuntary absence of food for a prolonged period, often leading to severe health consequences. Fasting, on the other hand, is a conscious, controlled decision to refrain from eating for specific windows of time. The intention? To allow our bodies to tap into stored energy (fat) and initiate processes like autophagy (remember that cellular tidying-up?).

**Myth 4: Fasting will eat away my muscles**

The imagery of fasting 'eating away' at our muscles can be downright terrifying. But let's unravel this: when our bodies enter a fasting state, they first use up glycogen. Once that's spent, they tap into stored fat, turning it into ketones for energy. Muscles? They're not the body's first choice for energy. And get this, fasting can also increase levels of a hormone called human growth hormone (HGH), which plays a vital role in muscle growth and maintenance.

**Myth 5: Women shouldn't fast; it's harmful**

This one's particularly close to our hearts. Yes, women's bodies are uniquely sensitive to caloric intake, primarily because of our reproductive role. But this doesn't mean women can't benefit from fasting. It simply means our approach might be different. It's all about listening to our bodies and making informed, gentle decisions, which we'll explore deeper in the coming chapters.

**Myth 6: Fasting is too hard; I'll always be hungry**

I hear you. The idea of not eating for extended periods can sound daunting. But here's the fascinating thing: hunger is not just a linear increase with time. It comes in waves, governed by our hunger hormone, ghrelin. With consistent fasting, many people find their hunger levels actually stabilize, and those intense pangs diminish. It's like training a muscle – it gets easier with practice.

**Myth 7: I can eat whatever I want in my eating window**

While intermittent fasting isn't super prescriptive about what to eat, it doesn't hand us a free ticket to junk food land. The goal is holistic health, right? So, it's essential to focus on balanced, nutritious meals. Think of it as fueling your body with the best, high-octane fuel to keep it purring like a well-tuned car.

**Myth 8: Fasting will make me less productive and more tired**

Initially, as your body adjusts, you might feel a dip in energy. But, and this is the exciting part, many who practice intermittent fasting report increased energy levels and sharper focus once they're past the adjustment phase. Why? Ketones (from fat breakdown) are a potent fuel source for the brain!

**Myth 9: Intermittent fasting is a one-size-fits-all approach**

Absolutely not! Just as we have our unique style, quirks, and preferences, our fasting journey should be tailored to fit us perfectly. There are various fasting protocols, and part of this journey is finding the one that syncs harmoniously with our lifestyle, body, and goals.

**Myth 10: You can't exercise while fasting**

Quite the contrary! Exercising during a fasted state can amplify fat burning and boost metabolic health. However, the key is to listen to your body. Some might prefer light workouts, while others feel great doing more intense sessions. It's all about finding your rhythm.

In conclusion, like any journey, there will always be naysayers and myths clouding the path. But with every myth we dispel, we're one step closer to embracing the real, transformative power of intermittent fasting. Remember, dear reader, knowledge is not just power, but it's also freedom – freedom from misconceptions, and freedom to make the best choices for our unique selves. Onward we go!

# Chapter 1: Introduction to Intermittent Fasting
## Part III: Women and Fasting: A Unique Perspective

As we travel deeper into the realm of intermittent fasting, it's essential to address a topic close to my heart – and likely yours too. While the fundamental principles of fasting apply to all, the female body, with its beautiful complexities and rhythms, interacts with fasting in its own distinct ways. So, let's embark on this enlightening voyage, hand in hand, exploring how fasting uniquely influences women.

### The Dance of Hormones

It's a dance that's been happening since time immemorial. A dance that shapes our lives in ways we often can't even fathom. I'm talking about the delicate ballet of female hormones. Estrogen, progesterone, and others are the lead performers, influencing everything from our menstrual cycles to mood swings.

Fasting can affect these hormones, but it's not a one-way street. For example, short-term fasting may boost estrogen levels, enhancing cognitive function and mood. But, an extended fast might disrupt the menstrual cycle in some women. It's a balance, and understanding these nuances ensures our fasting journey aligns with our body's rhythm.

### The Monthly Cycle and Fasting

Every month, our body embarks on a hormonal roller-coaster, gracefully transitioning through different phases of the menstrual cycle. And here's the fascinating bit: our body's response to fasting can vary depending on the phase!

- **Follicular Phase (Day 1-14):** This phase starts on the first day of menstruation and lasts until ovulation. It's characterized by a rise in estrogen. During this phase, many women find they can fast with more ease and experience increased energy.

- **Luteal Phase (Day 15-28):** Post ovulation, progesterone levels rise, preparing the body for a potential pregnancy. Some women might feel hungrier during this phase, making extended fasts a bit more challenging. It's essential to be kind to ourselves and adapt our fasting schedules if needed.

**The Power of Metabolism**

Women are incredible. Our bodies are designed to bear and nurture life, and that comes with a metabolism that's adept at storing energy efficiently. While this was a survival boon in ancient times, in today's world of abundant calories, it can be a challenge.

Fasting offers a way to recalibrate, allowing us to tap into stored fat more effectively. However, women might experience a slightly slower metabolic boost from fasting compared to men. But slow and steady wins the race, right? It's all about patience and celebrating every victory, no matter how small.

**Pregnancy, Breastfeeding, and Fasting**

Navigating the waters of pregnancy and breastfeeding is a journey filled with joy, anticipation, and, yes, a dash of apprehension. Nutrition during these periods is paramount. If you're pregnant or breastfeeding, fasting might not be ideal. The body needs consistent energy, and there's an increased demand for nutrients. Always consult with a healthcare professional before making any decisions.

**Menopause and Beyond**

Ah, menopause. A time of transition, of saying goodbye to one phase and embracing the blossoming of another. Hormonal changes during menopause can lead to weight gain, especially around the midsection. Here's the silver lining: intermittent fasting can be a powerful tool during this period. It can help manage weight, enhance mood, and even alleviate some menopausal symptoms.

However, as bone density can be a concern for post-menopausal women, it's essential to ensure adequate calcium and vitamin D intake. Once again, always tailor your fasting journey to your unique needs, and don't hesitate to seek guidance.

**Stress, Cortisol, and the Female Body**

Let's talk about stress. Our bodies react to fasting as a form of mild stress, releasing the hormone cortisol. Now, in small doses, cortisol is beneficial. But, given the myriad of stresses modern women face, from juggling work to family responsibilities, it's essential to be mindful. If you're going through a particularly stressful phase, you might want to reconsider the timing and duration of your fasts.

Dearest reader, the relationship between women and fasting is profound, intricate, and deeply personal. Our bodies are temples of transformation, adapting and evolving through each life phase. Fasting is a tool, a way to honor and support these transitions. Remember, it's not about stringent rules but about harmony, listening to your body, and adapting with grace. The journey ahead will be filled with learning, self-discovery, and moments of profound clarity. I can't wait to explore it with you.

# CHAPTER 2: EVOLUTIONARY BASIS FOR FASTING

## Part I: History of Women's Eating Patterns

Ah, the tapestry of time! As we delve into the history of women's eating patterns, we're not just looking back through decades or centuries. We're traveling millennia back, tracing the footsteps of our earliest ancestors, understanding how they ate and why. And it's quite the tale! So, let's hop onto our metaphorical time machines and journey into the vast expanse of human history.

**In the Days of Hunters and Gatherers**

Long before supermarkets lined our streets and takeouts became a click away, our foremothers were part of nomadic tribes, living as hunters and gatherers. Imagine this: vast landscapes, untamed wilderness, and the eternal quest for food.

In these times, consistency was a luxury. Women played a pivotal role as gatherers, collecting berries, nuts, roots, and occasionally hunting smaller animals. The food wasn't always plentiful. There were days of abundance and days of scarcity. This natural ebb and flow meant that our ancient sisters often went extended periods without food, their bodies becoming adept at utilizing stored energy efficiently. It wasn't called "intermittent fasting" back then—it was simply survival.

## The Dawn of Agriculture

Fast forward a few millennia, and the landscape changed. With the advent of agriculture, around 10,000 years ago, humans began to settle. Women, once wanderers, now had a fixed abode. They began cultivating land, planting seeds, and reaping harvests.

While this ensured a more consistent food supply, it wasn't always year-round. There were still seasons of plenty and seasons of want. Harvest time brought grains, fruits, and vegetables in abundance. But winter? It often meant leaner times, mirroring those fasting periods of old. Our ancestral women had to be strategic, storing food, and again, sometimes going without, their bodies gracefully adapting to these patterns.

## Medieval Times to the Renaissance

As societies grew more complex, so did women's roles. They were caregivers, healers, and often the ones preparing meals. Seasons still dictated food availability. Women of this era knew the art of preservation—salting meats, pickling vegetables, and fermenting.

Yet, fasting took on a new dimension here. It wasn't just about food scarcity anymore. Religious and cultural practices began to incorporate fasting. For many women, fasting became a spiritual endeavor—a time to connect with the divine, seek penance, or introspect. Their bodies, minds, and souls intertwined in this ritual.

## Victorian Era to Early 20th Century

Ah, the age of corsets, etiquette, and afternoon teas! But behind the elegance of the Victorian era, there were also societal pressures. The 'ideal' feminine figure was celebrated, often leading women to adopt restrictive diets.

Then came the war years of the early 20th century. Food rationing became a reality in many parts of the world. Women, while contributing to the war effort, were also managing households on limited resources. Their resilience, creativity, and adaptability shone through as they navigated these challenging times.

**Modern Era and Today**

The late 20th and 21st centuries have seen unprecedented changes. Food is now available around the clock, and for many, it's abundant. The challenge today is not the scarcity of food but its overabundance. Fast food, processed meals, and snacks galore!

However, amidst this plenty, many women feel a disconnection. The ancient rhythms, the dance with nature, seems lost. This is where intermittent fasting comes in, offering a bridge, a way to reconnect with those age-old patterns. It's not just about weight loss or health; it's also about rediscovering a rhythm that's been part of women's history for eons.

Reflecting on this journey, it's evident: the history of women's eating patterns is a testament to adaptability, resilience, and evolution. From the vast plains of prehistoric Earth to the bustling cities of today, women have navigated changing landscapes, their bodies gracefully adapting to different eating patterns.

As we embrace intermittent fasting, we're not just adopting a new health regimen. We're tapping into an age-old legacy, a shared history that courses through our veins. It's a beautiful reminder that as women, we carry the strength, wisdom, and adaptability of countless generations before us. What a powerful legacy to honor and continue!

# Chapter 2: Evolutionary Basis for Fasting
## Part II: The Hunter-Gatherer Legacy

Sit tight, dear reader, because we're about to embark on a journey back in time—a journey that's less about time-traveling and more about understanding the intrinsic relationship we, especially as women, share with our hunter-gatherer ancestors.

### Walking in Their Shoes

Picture this: vast expanses of untouched nature, the sound of leaves rustling, and perhaps the distant call of a bird. In this world, the supermarket is the forest, the savannah, the rivers, and the coastlines. The aisles are the meandering paths tread by our ancient sisters, searching, seeking, and often waiting for their next meal.

These women didn't have the luxury of popping into a store for a quick snack or grabbing a latte when they felt like it. Their lives revolved around finding food, which was sporadic and unpredictable. They had to be in tune with nature's cycles, understanding when berries would ripen or when fish would be abundant.

### Fasting Wasn't a Choice; It Was a Way of Life

For our hunter-gatherer foremothers, fasting wasn't about a trendy diet or a detox after a weekend binge. It was often a necessity. With inconsistent food supplies, there were times they had plenty, and then there were times when they had very little.

This inconsistency wired their bodies—and by extension, ours—in a remarkable way. When food was abundant, their bodies stored energy, and during lean periods, they efficiently used these energy reserves. They didn't call it intermittent fasting. It was simply living, adapting, and thriving.

### The Social Fabric of Hunter-Gatherer Women

Now, let's debunk a common myth. When we think of hunter-gatherers, we often envision men hunting mammoths. But women played an equally vital role, often bringing in a substantial part of the tribe's food.

Women worked in collaboration, foraging for nuts, seeds, plants, and even hunting smaller animals. These outings were more than just food quests; they were social occasions, moments of bonding, sharing knowledge, and weaving a tapestry of communal stories.

Through these shared endeavors, women didn't just feed their tribes; they nurtured connections, building strong social networks that were essential for survival. This legacy of community and collaboration is still alive within us. When women come together, magic happens—even if it's over a shared meal rather than a hunt!

**Adaptable Bodies and Minds**

Our hunter-gatherer ancestors, especially the women, were masters of adaptability. Think about it: they navigated changing seasons, unpredictable weather, and varying food sources. Their strength wasn't just physical; it was deeply mental and emotional.

These women developed keen instincts, acute observational skills, and a profound understanding of nature's rhythms. Their bodies, too, mirrored this adaptability, evolving mechanisms to cope with food scarcity. This metabolic flexibility is a gift handed down through generations, one that many of us are now tapping into through intermittent fasting.

**Tapping Into Our Primal Rhythms**

So, why does the hunter-gatherer legacy matter in our modern world, filled with skyscrapers, digital devices, and 24/7 food availability? Because, deep down, our biological rhythms still resonate with those of our ancestors.

In our contemporary lives, where food is often overabundant and always on-demand, we've lost touch with these primal rhythms. We eat not just when we're hungry, but often out of boredom, stress, or societal cues. But the beauty of intermittent fasting is that it allows us to reconnect with these ancient rhythms, to listen to our bodies' signals, and to eat in harmony with our evolutionary legacy.

As we wrap up this part of our journey, take a moment to reflect. Our lineage is embedded with stories of resilience, adaptability, and strength. The hunter-gatherer legacy is not a tale of the past; it's a narrative that lives within us, shaping our instincts, our appetites, and our approach to food.

By understanding and honoring this legacy, we don't just adopt a dietary pattern; we embrace a holistic way of life that respects our history, our biology, and our innate need for community. And in this embrace, we find a sense of belonging, a connection to the vast web of life, and a roadmap for nourishing not just our bodies, but our souls too.

# Chapter 2: Evolutionary Basis for Fasting
# Part III: Modern-Day Implications

Ah, the modern world. It's a far cry from the days of vast savannahs and thick forests where our foremothers wandered. Today, we have climate-controlled homes, instant communication, and yes, 24/7 access to food from around the world. With all this progress, it's only natural to wonder, "How does our ancient past impact us in this fast-paced, tech-driven age?" Let's dive deep into this confluence of ancient biology and contemporary lifestyles.

**Feast or Famine in a World of Plenty**

Our hunter-gatherer ancestors lived in a world of unpredictability, where periods of feasting could swiftly turn to times of famine. Their bodies, remarkably adaptable, learned to harness energy and store it for the not-so-plentiful days. Today, we find ourselves in an unusual situation where, for many, it's an almost perpetual feast. The once beneficial trait of storing excess energy has, in our calorie-rich environment, laid the groundwork for modern health concerns like obesity, type 2 diabetes, and heart diseases.

**Lost Rhythms in a 24/7 World**

Remember the beautiful rhythms our ancestors danced to? Following the sun's rise and set, they rested and rose with nature. Today, in our world of bright screens and night shifts, many of us have become disconnected from these natural cycles. With late-night snacking and irregular meal timings, our internal clocks (or circadian rhythms) are often thrown out of whack. There's growing evidence suggesting that eating in sync with our body's natural rhythms can be beneficial for our metabolism, sleep, and overall well-being.

**The Stress Connection**

While we're no longer hunting for our next meal or avoiding

predators, the modern world has its set of stressors. From looming deadlines to financial worries, stress is a constant for many. Evolutionarily, stress signaled a threat. In response, our bodies would store fat, anticipating the need for extra energy.

Fast-forward to today, chronic stress, even if it's not from a physical threat, can still trigger this ancient response. Pair this with readily available high-calorie foods, and it becomes clear how our evolutionary traits, beneficial in the past, might be contributing to our contemporary health challenges.

**The Power of Intermittent Fasting**

So, where does intermittent fasting fit into this modern narrative? By mimicking the natural feast and famine cycles, intermittent fasting can help realign our bodies with those primal rhythms. It allows our system to tap into stored energy, giving our digestive system a break and promoting cellular repair. In many ways, it's like hitting the reset button, aligning ourselves more closely with how our bodies have evolved to function.

**Harnessing Our Legacy for Today**

The beauty of understanding our evolutionary past is that it equips us to make informed decisions about our health today. While we can't turn back the clock and live like our hunter-gatherer ancestors (and honestly, who would give up modern comforts!), we can adopt practices that respect our biology.

This isn't about romanticizing the past but about realizing that our bodies have a built-in wisdom. By honoring this wisdom —whether it's through intermittent fasting, prioritizing sleep, or managing stress—we can navigate the modern world with grace, health, and vitality.

**The Community Aspect**

One of the most potent lessons from our ancestors is the

power of community. While the context has changed, our need for connection remains. Women, historically and even now, thrive in communal settings. Sharing our fasting journeys, be it challenges or triumphs, with a supportive community can make the process more enjoyable and sustainable. Remember, it's not just about individual goals; it's about collective well-being.

As we stand at this crossroads of ancient legacies and modern challenges, there's a profound opportunity for transformation. Our evolutionary history isn't just a tale of survival; it's a testament to adaptability. In understanding and respecting this, we can craft a life that marries the best of both worlds—the ancient wisdom of our foremothers and the advancements of today.

In our hands, we hold the power to shape our health, drawing from the deep well of ancestral wisdom and applying it to the unique challenges and opportunities of the present. It's a journey of rediscovery, of reconnection, and most importantly, of reclaiming our inherent strength and vitality. So, as we move forward, let's do so with gratitude for our past and excitement for the possibilities ahead.

# CHAPTER 3: THE FEMALE PHYSIOLOGY & FASTING

## Part I: The Menstrual Cycle and Fasting

As we step into this chapter, we're venturing into a topic deeply personal and intimate to every woman: our menstrual cycle. This cyclical rhythm, though often associated with periods alone, encompasses so much more. It's a dance of hormones, emotions, and energy levels. And as we discuss fasting, understanding this unique ebb and flow becomes vital. Let's delve into the intricate relationship between fasting and our menstrual cycle.

**Understanding the Menstrual Symphony**

First things first, let's acquaint ourselves with the key players in this hormonal symphony: estrogen and progesterone. Estrogen usually dominates the first half of the cycle, leading up to ovulation. It's like the uplifting crescendo in music, boosting mood, energy, and even our metabolism. Progesterone, on the other hand, takes center stage post-ovulation, calming things down, promoting relaxation and nesting instincts.

So, what does this have to do with fasting? Well, everything!

**Fasting in the First Half of the Cycle**

Given the naturally elevated energy levels due to rising estrogen in the first half of the cycle (the follicular phase), many women find it easier to fast during this time. The body is more insulin-sensitive, which means it's more efficient at using carbs for energy. As a result, hunger pangs might be less pronounced, and you might even experience increased mental clarity.

But there's a caveat. Around ovulation, our hunger might surge due to a brief testosterone spike. It's nature's way of saying, "Hey, it's prime baby-making time!" So, if you find yourself ravenous around ovulation, it's perfectly normal. Listen to your body and adjust your fasting window if needed.

**Navigating the Second Half of the Cycle**

The luteal phase, the second half of the cycle after ovulation, can be a different ball game. As progesterone levels rise, you might notice a drop in energy. You're more insulin resistant, which means you might crave carbs. These are signs from our body, preparing for a potential pregnancy.

Fasting during this phase can be a tad more challenging. The increased carb cravings aren't just in your head; they're rooted in physiology. If you're practicing intermittent fasting and find it tough during the luteal phase, consider shortening your fasting window or incorporating more nutrient-dense carbs during your eating window.

**The Menstrual Phase: To Fast or Not to Fast?**

When Aunt Flo visits, many women wonder whether it's wise to fast. Now, there's no one-size-fits-all answer. Some women find fasting during their period very natural and comfortable, perhaps because the body is already in a detoxifying mode. Others might feel an increased need for nourishment, given the energy expended in shedding the uterine lining.

Here's the golden rule: Listen to your body. If fasting feels right, go ahead. If not, give yourself grace. Remember, intermittent fasting is a tool, not a strict regimen. It's meant to fit into your life, not the other way around.

**The Emotional Landscape**

Our menstrual cycle isn't just a physiological phenomenon; it's an emotional journey. Many women report heightened emotions or increased introspection during certain phases. Recognizing and honoring these shifts is crucial when incorporating fasting. On days when emotions run high, the added stress of a strict fasting window might not be ideal. And that's okay. Emotional well-being is as crucial as physical health.

**Tailoring Fasting to Your Cycle**

Harnessing the knowledge of your cycle can allow you to tailor your fasting regimen in harmony with your body's natural rhythms. It's like riding the waves, leveraging the highs, and supporting the lows. By aligning with your cycle, you're not just optimizing the benefits of fasting, but you're also practicing self-care, tuning into your body's whispers (or sometimes, loud declarations!).

In essence, the relationship between our menstrual cycle and fasting is profound and deeply personal. It's a dance of intuition, understanding, and adaptability. As women, our strength lies in our ability to ebb and flow, to adapt, and to nourish ourselves—body, mind, and soul. As we journey through the world of fasting, let's remember to honor this intrinsic rhythm, celebrating the beauty, wisdom, and resilience of our female physiology.

## Chapter 3: The Female Physiology & Fasting
## Part II: Hormones and Hunger

As we navigate the seas of intermittent fasting, understanding our internal compass — hormones — is crucial. It's almost poetic, isn't it? How these tiny molecules, invisible to our eyes, steer our hunger, energy, moods, and so much more. So, let's unravel this intricate dance between our hormones and the sensation of hunger.

### Hormones: The Maestros of Metabolism

Before we dive into specific hormones, let's appreciate the broader picture. Hormones, in essence, are our body's communication system. Imagine them as messengers, zipping around, ensuring that our organs are in harmony. When it comes to hunger, a few hormones play leading roles.

### 1. Leptin & Ghrelin: The Yin and Yang

Often dubbed the 'hunger hormones', leptin and ghrelin work in tandem. While leptin sends the "I'm full" signal, ghrelin is the one nudging you, saying, "Hey, time to eat!"

When you fast, or even when you just reduce calorie intake, ghrelin levels rise, making you feel hungrier. Over time, with consistent fasting, the body adapts, and these ghrelin surges diminish. Leptin, on the other hand, is released from fat cells and signals satiety. But here's the kicker: if we have higher levels of body fat, and by extension, higher levels of leptin, our brain might become 'leptin resistant', making us feel perpetually hungry. This is where intermittent fasting can be a game-changer. By improving our sensitivity to these hormones, fasting can recalibrate our hunger cues.

### 2. Insulin: Not Just About Sugar

Ah, insulin. While primarily known for its role in regulating blood sugar, it plays a pivotal part in hunger too. When we eat, especially carbs, our blood sugar rises, prompting insulin's release. Insulin ensures our cells get the glucose they need for energy. Consistently high insulin levels, however, can desensitize our cells to it, leading to insulin resistance. This not only paves the way for type 2 diabetes but also disrupts our hunger signals. Fasting, by giving our body breaks from insulin surges, can improve insulin sensitivity.

**3. Cortisol: The Stress Link**

Ever found yourself raiding the fridge when stressed? That's cortisol at play. This stress hormone, while essential in 'fight or flight' scenarios, can wreak havoc when chronically elevated. It stimulates glucose production, leading to increased insulin and subsequently, hunger. And if you're wondering why you crave sugary, fatty foods in stressful times, well, these foods dampen stress responses, making them 'comfort foods' in a real sense. Intermittent fasting, by modulating cortisol levels, can break this stress-hunger loop. But remember, if you're already under significant stress, diving straight into strict fasting might be counterproductive. Baby steps, dear reader.

**4. Estrogen: The Feminine Touch**

We touched upon estrogen earlier, but its link with hunger deserves special mention. Estrogen, especially mid-cycle, can suppress appetite. However, during periods or in conditions like polycystic ovary syndrome (PCOS) where estrogen balance is off-kilter, hunger and cravings can intensify. By supporting balanced insulin levels, intermittent fasting can indirectly influence estrogen balance and, in turn, hunger.

**Navigating Hormonal Hunger Waves**

Understanding these hormonal dynamics is empowering. It reminds us that hunger isn't just about an empty stomach; it's a symphony of signals. Some days, you might feel ravenous, and on others, surprisingly satiated. Instead of judging these fluctuations, can we embrace them as part of our beautifully complex system?

**Strategies to Harness Hormonal Hunger:**

**1. Stay Hydrated:** Sometimes, our bodies confuse thirst with hunger. Drinking water can help decipher this.

**2. Prioritize Sleep:** Lack of sleep can skew leptin and ghrelin balance, amplifying hunger. Rest up!

**3. Mindful Eating:** By tuning into our meals, we can better listen to our satiety signals.

**4. Balanced Meals:** Incorporate proteins, healthy fats, and complex carbs. They can stabilize blood sugar and provide sustained energy.

**5. Stress Management:** Find outlets like meditation, exercise, or journaling to manage stress, keeping cortisol in check.

In this waltz of hormones and hunger, there's wisdom, resilience, and fluidity. Intermittent fasting isn't about suppressing hunger but understanding and respecting it. It's about reconnecting with our bodies, discerning between physiological hunger and emotional or habitual eating. By understanding the hormonal cues, we can make informed, compassionate choices, aligning with our well-being goals. Here's to celebrating our hormonal orchestra and dancing in harmony with our hunger!

# Chapter 3: The Female Physiology & Fasting
## Part III: Impact on Metabolism

Oh, the illustrious metabolism! Haven't we all wished, at some point or another, that ours worked a bit more in our favor? You've likely heard stories of friends who can seemingly eat anything without gaining weight, attributing it to a 'fast metabolism.' So, let's pull back the curtain on this metabolic magic and understand how fasting impacts it, especially for us women.

### Deciphering Metabolism

To put it simply, metabolism is the sum of all chemical reactions in our bodies that keep us alive — from breaking down food for energy to repairing cells. Think of it as your body's engine, with the rate at which it burns fuel (calories) as the metabolic rate. Several factors influence this rate, including age, muscle mass, and yes, our hormones.

### Fasting and the Metabolic Flame

Fasting has a fascinating relationship with metabolism. Contrary to popular belief, short-term fasting might actually boost your metabolic rate. Surprised? It's a primordial response. Our ancestors, when faced with food scarcity, had to be alert and agile to hunt or gather food. So, the body, in its infinite wisdom, amped up the energy production.

However, prolonged fasting or extreme caloric restriction can backfire. The body, in an attempt to conserve energy, might slow down the metabolic rate. It's like switching to an energy-saving mode. This is where intermittent fasting shines. By cycling between eating and fasting periods, we might reap the benefits of a metabolic boost without the drawback of a slowdown.

### Women, Fasting, and Metabolism: A Delicate Balance

As women, our metabolic relationship with fasting is nuanced.

Hormones like estrogen influence how we store and burn fat. And let's not forget the significant metabolic shifts during different life phases: menstruation, pregnancy, postpartum, and menopause.

**1. Menstruation:** Ever felt hungrier during your periods? That's because our metabolic rate slightly rises pre-menstruation. Fasting during this time might be challenging, and that's okay. Listen to your body.

**2. Pregnancy & Postpartum:** Pregnancy is a metabolic marathon. The body is nurturing another human! Postpartum, the body is healing and possibly breastfeeding, which is energetically demanding. Extreme fasting might not be the best choice here, but gentle, shorter fasts, with medical guidance, could be considered.

**3. Menopause:** As estrogen levels drop, our metabolism naturally slows. The muscle mass might decrease, and fat storage patterns change. Fasting, combined with resistance training, can be a powerful duo during this phase, helping preserve muscle and boosting metabolic health.

**Thyroid Talk**

The thyroid gland is often dubbed the metabolic powerhouse. Thyroid hormones regulate our metabolic rate, energy levels, and more. Fasting impacts thyroid hormones, but here's where it gets tricky for women. Our thyroid function is closely linked with estrogen. Extreme fasting can reduce thyroid hormones, potentially slowing metabolism. So, a word of caution: if you have thyroid issues or symptoms, consult with a healthcare professional before embarking on fasting regimes.

**Metabolic Flexibility: The Real Goal**

Beyond just speeding up metabolism, fasting promotes something even more valuable: metabolic flexibility. It's the ability of our bodies to seamlessly switch between fuel sources, from glucose (from carbs) to ketones (from fats). Imagine a hybrid car, smoothly transitioning between fuel types based on the journey's demands. That's metabolic flexibility.

For us women, achieving this flexibility is empowering. It means reduced energy crashes, sustained energy, better fat burning, and improved hormonal balance. Intermittent fasting, by periodically depleting glucose stores, nudges the body to tap into fat reserves, enhancing this flexibility.

**Tailoring Your Fasting Approach**

While the metabolic benefits of fasting sound promising, the key lies in personalization. Our bodies, life stages, and daily demands are unique. Some might thrive on longer fasts, while others benefit from shorter, more frequent ones. It's a journey of self-discovery, of tuning in and adjusting based on our body's whispers (or sometimes, loud protests!).

**Final Thoughts on Metabolism and Fasting**

The metabolic realm is enchanting, with its ebbs and flows, its intricate dance with hormones and life phases. As we embrace intermittent fasting, let's shift our focus from merely 'boosting' metabolism to nurturing a responsive, flexible metabolic system. It's not about fitting into an old pair of jeans but fitting comfortably into our bodies, today and every day. Through understanding, patience, and a dash of metabolic magic, we can journey towards our best health. Remember, dear reader, your metabolic song is unique. Dance to its rhythm, and let the wonders of fasting be your dance partner.

# CHAPTER 4: COMMON FASTING PROTOCOLS

## Part I: The 16/8 Method

Let's dive into the world of fasting protocols, shall we? Picture this: It's like standing at the buffet of health, each dish promising unique flavors of wellness. And today, we're focusing on a crowd-favorite dish - the 16/8 method.

The 16/8 method, fondly known as the 'Leangains protocol' by some, sounds technical but is delightfully simple in essence. It requires you to fast for 16 hours and limit your eating to an 8-hour window. Think of it as a daily routine where the majority of your fasting happens when you're, well, catching your beauty sleep.

**Setting the Scene: Why 16/8?**

Before we delve into the details, let's ask: Why 16 hours? Is it a magic number? In truth, the magic lies in the balance it strikes. It's long enough to trigger some of the beneficial metabolic shifts we associate with fasting but short enough for most of us to manage without feeling overwhelmed. It's like the Goldilocks of fasting - not too short, not too long, just right.

**A Day in the Life on the 16/8 Plan**

Imagine this: You finish dinner at 7 pm. As you dive into your evening routine, reading, maybe some Netflix (no judgment here!), your body is gradually depleting its readily available energy source - glucose. As dawn breaks and you're still tucked in, dreaming away, your body shifts. It starts tapping into fat reserves for energy, producing ketones. By the time you're up and ready to seize the day, you're in a mild fat-burning mode, even if you don't feel radically different.

Your first meal? It might be at 11 am. A luscious brunch, if you will. From then, you'd eat your meals and snacks, listening to hunger cues, till 7 pm, after which the cycle begins again.

**Benefits of the 16/8 Dance**

**1. Simplicity:** No elaborate meal plans or calorie counting. The primary focus? Timing.

**2. Flexibility:** Choose your 8-hour window based on your lifestyle. Not a morning person? Maybe you prefer lunch at 1 pm and wrap up dinner by 9 pm. It's all about what feels right for you.

**3. Metabolic Shifts:** As mentioned, prolonged periods without food might encourage your body to tap into fat reserves. It's a gentle nudge towards metabolic flexibility.

**4. Gut Rest:** Giving your digestive system a break can be beneficial. Think of it as letting your inner housekeeping team do a thorough cleanup without constant interruptions.

**5. Mindful Eating:** When you have a limited window, you might become more aware of what you eat and why. It's an invitation to savor, appreciate, and nourish.

**But... What About Women?**

Aha! This is where it gets intriguing. As we've previously discussed, women's bodies are a symphony of hormones. While many women thrive on the 16/8 method, some nuances are worth noting.

**1. Hormonal Balance:** Fasting affects insulin, cortisol, and ghrelin (hunger hormone) levels. For most women, the 16/8 method strikes a balance, offering fasting benefits without causing hormonal havoc. But, if you have hormonal imbalances, tread with caution and consult a healthcare professional.

**2. Menstrual Cycle:** Some women find it beneficial to adjust fasting lengths based on their menstrual cycle. If you feel incredibly hungry or fatigued a few days before your period, it might be worth shortening your fast or skipping it.

**3. Stress & Sleep:** Stress and lack of sleep can affect cortisol levels. Combining this with fasting might be overwhelming for some women. If you're going through a particularly stressful period or not catching enough zzz's, consider easing into fasting.

**Tips & Tricks for Rocking the 16/8**

**1. Stay Hydrated:** During your fasting window, water, herbal teas, and black coffee (in moderation) can be your companions.

**2. Prioritize Quality:** Just because it's an 8-hour eating window doesn't mean it's a junk food free-for-all. Prioritize whole, nutritious foods to nourish your body.

**3. Listen to Your Body:** Feel like 16 hours is a bit too much? It's okay to start with 14 and gradually work your way up.

**4. Consistency Over Perfection:** Missed a day? Had to break your fast early? It's alright. One day doesn't define your health journey. Pick up the rhythm the next day.

In the realm of intermittent fasting, the 16/8 method is like a gentle waltz. It's rhythmic, balanced, and can be tailored to your unique song. As you consider this dance, remember it's about more than just hours and food. It's about rediscovering a harmonious relationship with your body, understanding its rhythms, and dancing in sync. So, are you ready to take the floor?

# Chapter 4: Common Fasting Protocols
## Part II: The 5:2 Diet

Ah, the 5:2 Diet. It has an almost poetic ring to it, doesn't it? If you're envisioning a strict, complex regimen, I've got a pleasant surprise for you. The 5:2 Diet, sometimes called the 'Fast Diet', is one of the most approachable fasting methods out there. Let's uncover the beauty of this rhythm together.

**Understanding the 5:2 Beat**

Let's simplify this: for five days of the week, you eat without any specific calorie restrictions—your usual, balanced meals. The other two days? You reduce your caloric intake, typically to about 500-600 calories. These two days are known as your "fasting days." And guess what? They don't have to be consecutive.

Here's the delightful part: this isn't about starving or denying yourself. It's about recalibrating and giving your body a gentle rest.

**A Glimpse Into A 5:2 Week**

Let's walk through a typical week, shall we?

**Monday:** Your usual meals, listening to your hunger and fullness cues.
**Tuesday:** A light day—maybe a hearty soup for lunch and a salad with lean protein for dinner.
**Wednesday:** Back to your regular eating rhythm.
**Thursday:** Regular eating continues.
**Friday:** Another light day, perhaps a smoothie in the morning, and a grilled fish with veggies for dinner.
**Weekend:** You indulge in your regular meals, maybe even that slice of cake you've been eyeing!

The beauty of the 5:2 is its flexibility. Your fasting days can be any days you choose, as long as there are five regular eating days and two reduced-calorie days in your week.

**Why the 5:2 Resonates with So Many**

**1. Flexibility Galore:** Got a birthday party on Friday? No worries, shift your fasting day. This adaptability makes the 5:2 so sustainable and compatible with real life.

**2. Manageable Challenge:** For many, reducing calories for two days feels achievable, like a short sprint in the grand marathon of the week.

**3. Digestive Rest:** Like our previous protocols, the reduced-calorie days can offer your gut a break, helping with digestion and even reducing bloating.

**4. Metabolic Perks:** On your reduced-calorie days, your body might tap into those fat stores for energy, aiding weight management and metabolic health.

**A Special Note for the Ladies**

You guessed it! Our female physiology adds a layer of nuance to every fasting method, and the 5:2 is no exception.

**1. Caloric Considerations:** The often-cited 500-600 calorie range might not suit all. Some women, especially those very active, might fare better on 700-800 calories on their reduced days. The key? Listen to your body.

**2. Nutrient Density:** On your low-calorie days, it's crucial to get a bang for your buck. Opt for foods rich in nutrients. Think leafy greens, lean proteins, healthy fats like avocados, and fiber-filled veggies.

**3. Menstrual Cycle Awareness:** Some women find fasting during certain phases of their cycle, especially around menstruation, a bit challenging. If you're one of them, consider adjusting your fasting days to suit your cycle.

**Navigating Your 5:2 Journey with Grace**

**1. Hydration is Key:** Especially on your reduced-calorie days, ensure you're sipping water, herbal teas, or even broths to stay hydrated.

**2. Prioritize Protein and Fiber:** These can help keep you full. A spinach and chicken salad, a lentil soup, or a chia seed pudding can be your best friends on fasting days.

**3. Mindful Eating:** On both regular and fasting days, take a moment to savor your food. Chew slowly, relish the flavors, and notice how food nourishes you.

**4. Stay Active, but Sensibly:** On fasting days, you might want to swap high-intensity workouts for gentler activities like walking or yoga.

**5. Consult Before Diving In:** If you have medical conditions or are on medications, it's essential to consult with a healthcare professional before embracing the 5:2.

The 5:2 diet isn't about drastic measures; it's about balance. It's the gentle ebb and flow of the tide, the rhythm of inhaling and exhaling. And as with every fasting protocol, remember, it's not about perfection. It's about the journey, the learning, the syncing up with your body's needs. As you contemplate this dance of 5:2, know that it's another tool in your kit, a potential step towards harmony in health and spirit. So, ready to groove to this beat?

## Chapter 4: Common Fasting Protocols
## Part III: Alternate-Day Fasting

I can almost sense your curiosity bubbling as we embark on the next protocol: Alternate-Day Fasting (ADF). And, believe me, I felt the same way when I first stumbled upon it! Let's delve into this intriguing, age-old practice, pulling apart the myths, embracing the truths, and understanding if it could be the rhythm your body has been yearning for.

**The Dance of ADF**

Imagine for a moment a pendulum, swinging gracefully from one side to the other. That's Alternate-Day Fasting in a nutshell. On one day, you consume your regular meals without restriction. On the next, you significantly limit your caloric intake or, for some, abstain from calories entirely. And then? Well, you swing back to a day of regular eating. It's a dance of nourishment and rest, consumption and rejuvenation.

**A Day in the Life of ADF**

So, what might this look like in your day-to-day?

**Monday:** A typical day of nourishing meals.
**Tuesday:** A fasting day, perhaps with a light broth or a few pieces of fruit, staying below 500 calories. Or for the brave-hearted, a full fast with no calories, just hydration.
**Wednesday:** Back to feasting, savoring your meals, and relishing every bite.
**Thursday:** Another fasting or reduced-calorie day, and so on.

Notice that this isn't about deprivation, but rhythm—a cyclical journey that mirrors the natural ebb and flow of life.

**Why ADF Resonates with Some**

**1. Clear Boundaries:** There's something refreshing about the clarity of ADF. It's either a day you're eating regularly or a day you're fasting. No in-betweens, no gray areas.

**2. Promising Health Benefits:** Some studies suggest that ADF can support weight management, promote heart health, and even aid in blood sugar control.

**3. Flexibility:** If you find a particular fasting day challenging, you know the very next day allows you to eat normally. It's a short commitment, one day at a time.

**4. Spiritual & Mental Clarity:** Some find that on fasting days, without the focus on meals, there's a newfound clarity and space for reflection.

## The Female Touch: Navigating ADF as a Woman

Being women, we come with our unique set of challenges and gifts. And when it comes to ADF, our female physiology does throw in a few curveballs.

**1. Hormonal Balance:** The dance of our hormones means that some days we might feel naturally hungrier, especially around our menstrual cycle. It's okay to modify your ADF routine during these times.

**2. Listening to Your Body:** Some days, a full fast might feel right. Other times, a reduced-calorie day might be more in tune with your body's needs. It's all about tuning in.

**3. Nutrient Density:** Especially on fasting days when you do consume some calories, make them count! Think nutrient-rich, wholesome foods that offer sustenance.

**4. Activity Levels:** On fasting days, consider dialing back on strenuous activities. Gentle walks, stretching, or yoga can be excellent choices.

## Graceful Steps for ADF Success

**1. Stay Hydrated:** Especially on fasting days, hydration is crucial. Herbal teas, broths, or simply water can be your best companions.

**2. Plan Ahead:** Anticipate your fasting days. If you know you have a physically demanding or stressful day ahead, consider adjusting your fasting schedule.

**3. Community Support:** Share your ADF journey with a friend or join a group. It's always more comforting knowing someone else is dancing the same dance.

**4. Check In with a Professional:** If you're considering diving deep into ADF, especially the full fasting version, it's wise to consult a healthcare professional.

Alternate-Day Fasting isn't a one-size-fits-all solution. And while some swear by the mental clarity and health benefits it provides, others might find a different fasting protocol more suited to their lifestyle and physiological needs.

So, dear reader, as we swing this pendulum together, remember that it's all about finding harmony. The joy of ADF is in its rhythm, its clear demarcations, and the promise of renewal with each new day. Whether it's a dance you wish to join or simply appreciate from the sidelines, know that every step, every swing, is a move towards understanding and nurturing your unique self.

# CHAPTER 5: FASTING AND WEIGHT LOSS FOR WOMEN

## Part I: The Science of Weight Loss

Welcome to a chapter that's undoubtedly a hot topic for many. Weight loss. Those two words alone can conjure up a plethora of emotions - hope, anxiety, curiosity, maybe even skepticism. Whether you've been on countless weight loss journeys or are merely curious, let's take a moment to understand the science behind it. Because once you grasp the 'why', the 'how' becomes an easier path to navigate.

**Weight Loss: Not Just Calories In, Calories Out**

You've likely heard the mantra: "Eat fewer calories than you burn, and you'll lose weight." While it has its truths, it's also a gross simplification of a complex symphony of processes that occur in our bodies.

**1. Metabolism**: Think of it as the engine that burns the fuel (calories) we provide. Everyone's metabolic rate varies, influenced by factors like genetics, age, muscle mass, and more.

**2. Hormonal Regulation:** Hormones play a pivotal role in our hunger cues and where our bodies store fat. Leptin and ghrelin, for instance, are the hunger management duo, signaling when we're full or famished.

**3. Nutrient Absorption:** Not all calories are created equal. 100 calories from a candy bar and 100 calories from a handful of nuts have vastly different effects on our bodies, from how they're digested to the nutrients they offer.

## How Does Fasting Fit Into the Equation?

When you eat, your body spends hours processing that food, burning what it can from what you've consumed. This is especially true for carbohydrates (our primary energy source), which are converted into glucose. Any excess glucose gets stored as fat.

However, after a certain period without food (fasting), your body runs out of glucose to run on. This is when it flips the switch and starts burning stored fat for energy, a state called ketosis.

## Insulin: The Key Player

One hormone deserves special mention here: insulin. Whenever we eat, our bodies release insulin to help absorb the nutrients from our bloodstream. One of its primary jobs is to manage glucose levels. In the context of weight loss, the crucial point is this: high levels of insulin can prevent fat burning. By eating all the time, we maintain elevated insulin levels, which could hinder our weight loss goals.

Fasting provides a break, allowing insulin levels to drop, signaling the body to start burning stored fat.

## Women, Fat Storage, and Evolution

Diving deeper into the realm of females and weight loss, it's essential to recognize our evolutionary background. Historically, women have been the bearers of life. Our bodies, in preparation for potential pregnancies, are naturally inclined to store fat more efficiently than men, especially around the hips and thighs. This evolutionary trait ensured a steady energy reserve for both mother and child.

Fasting, for women, can be a tool to tap into these reserves, but it's crucial to approach it with an understanding of our evolutionary predisposition. That's why weight loss can sometimes seem more challenging for women, but it's not impossible.

**The Emotional and Psychological Layer**

Science isn't just about hormones and metabolic rates. Our relationship with food, body image, and self-worth plays a significant role in weight loss. Emotional eating, stress-induced snacking, or even societal pressures can influence our weight. Understanding and addressing these underlying issues is just as crucial as any dietary or exercise regimen.

**Benefits Beyond the Scale**

While weight loss might be a driving factor for many, fasting offers a myriad of benefits beyond just shedding pounds:

**1. Cellular Repair and Autophagy:** In a fasted state, cells initiate a waste removal process called autophagy. This involves breaking down and metabolizing broken and dysfunctional proteins that build up inside cells over time.

**2. Brain Health:** Fasting boosts the production of brain-derived neurotrophic factor (BDNF), which aids brain function and reduces the risk of neurodegenerative diseases.

**3. Improved Insulin Sensitivity:** Regular fasting can help lower blood sugar levels, reducing the risk of type 2 diabetes.

**4. Heart Health:** Fasting can improve numerous risk factors for cardiovascular diseases, such as blood pressure, cholesterol levels, triglycerides, and inflammatory markers.

**Navigating Weight Loss as a Woman**

While the science is universal, each woman's journey is

personal. Remember, dear reader, that you're more than a number on a scale. Celebrate the small victories, the non-scale ones like more energy, clearer skin, better sleep, and enhanced mood. Seek a holistic approach that blends the science with self-love, patience, and perseverance.

As we dive deeper into this chapter, let's keep this foundation in mind: weight loss is a dance of physiology, psychology, and emotion. Understanding the science is the first step, but listening to your body and honoring your unique journey is equally essential.

# Chapter 5: Fasting and Weight Loss for Women
## Part II: The Role of Insulin

Ah, insulin. If there was ever a character in the intricate drama of our body's functions that deserved its own spotlight, it's this little hormone. But why, you ask? Well, dear reader, you're about to embark on a fascinating journey that'll not only demystify this enigmatic actor but also underscore its pivotal role in our health, particularly in the realm of weight loss.

### Insulin 101: The Basics

Before we delve deep, let's start with the basics. Picture insulin as the body's principal doorkeeper. When we consume food, especially carbohydrates, our body breaks them down into a type of sugar called glucose, which then enters the bloodstream. Now, glucose is a source of energy, but it needs to be transported into our cells to be used. And who does that? Our doorkeeper, insulin.

Every time we eat, the pancreas releases insulin, which then unlocks our cells, allowing glucose to enter and be used as fuel. The more we eat, especially sugary or carb-heavy meals, the more insulin is produced.

### Insulin's Dual Role: Storage and Regulation

Here's the catch. Insulin doesn't just help with energy regulation. It also plays a major role in storing excess glucose. When there's too much glucose in our bloodstream, insulin ensures it gets stored as fat for later use. Evolutionarily, this made sense. Our ancestors didn't have the luxury of 24/7 access to food. Storing excess energy as fat was a survival mechanism during times of scarcity.

However, in our modern world, where most of us have abundant access to food around the clock, this storage system, combined with constant eating, can lead to weight gain. The perpetual cycle of consuming carbs, releasing insulin, and storing fat becomes a routine.

## Hyperinsulinemia: The Overwhelmed System

In our carb-laden diets, where processed foods and sugars are rampant, our bodies often release more insulin than necessary. Over time, this constant flood of insulin can lead to a state called hyperinsulinemia, which means there are consistently high levels of insulin in the blood.

Hyperinsulinemia can become a significant roadblock for those trying to lose weight. How? With so much insulin in the bloodstream, the body is always in storage mode, making it challenging to burn stored fat.

## Insulin Resistance: Knocking on Closed Doors

There's another plot twist in our insulin saga: insulin resistance. Imagine knocking on a door repeatedly, but no one answers. That's what happens at a cellular level. Due to factors like obesity, a sedentary lifestyle, and, most importantly, a diet high in refined carbs and sugars, our cells become "resistant" to the effects of insulin. They stop responding.

This resistance means that the pancreas works overtime, producing even more insulin. It's a vicious cycle, as the more insulin we have in our system, the harder it becomes to burn fat, leading to more weight gain, which only exacerbates insulin resistance.

## Women, PCOS, and the Insulin Connection

For many women, insulin isn't just about weight. Polycystic ovary syndrome (PCOS), a prevalent condition, has a direct link with insulin resistance. Many women with PCOS often experience weight gain, and that's not a mere coincidence. The insulin resistance inherent in PCOS makes weight management a significant challenge.

## Fasting and Insulin: A Path to Sensitivity

Now, after all the intense drama, here's the silver lining: intermittent fasting. By reducing the eating window, we allow our bodies a break from producing insulin. This break helps reduce the overall levels of insulin in our bloodstream, pushing the body to start burning stored fat for energy.

Moreover, fasting can help improve insulin sensitivity over time. This means our cells respond better to insulin, requiring the pancreas to produce less, which can lead to better blood sugar control and more efficient fat burning.

## A Word of Caution

While understanding insulin is a massive step towards effective weight management, it's crucial to remember that everyone's body is unique. Fasting can be a useful tool, but it's vital to listen to your body and consult healthcare professionals, especially if you have underlying health conditions.

## To Conclude: A Newfound Respect for Insulin

Insulin is so much more than a biochemical reaction in our bodies. It's a protector, a regulator, and sometimes, when out of balance, a formidable foe. For women aiming to manage their weight, understanding the role of insulin can be life-changing.

So, as we progress further into our fasting journey, remember the lessons of insulin. It's not about vilifying it, but respecting its function, understanding its effects, and harnessing its power to serve our health goals. And with this knowledge, dear reader, you're one step closer to making informed choices on your health journey.

Chapter 5: Fasting and Weight Loss for Women
Part III: Sustainable Weight Loss

Alright, lovely readers, let's have a heart-to-heart. We've delved deep into the science of weight loss and decoded the pivotal role of insulin. But here's a truth bomb: understanding the science is just one side of the coin. The real challenge? Sustainability. Because, let's face it, how many times have we embarked on a weight loss journey, only to find ourselves back at square one after a few months, or worse, weeks?

The goal isn't just to shed those pounds; it's to keep them off. Sustainable weight loss is the key, and it's about more than just a number on the scale. It's about creating a lifestyle that feels right, is manageable, and, most importantly, is joyful. So, without further ado, let's dive into the world of sustainable weight loss.

**Understanding the Why**

First and foremost, let's talk motivation. Why do you want to lose weight? Is it societal pressure? A looming event? Or a genuine desire for better health? Your "why" is the foundation of your weight loss journey, and it has to be strong, personal, and authentic. It's the fire that will keep you going when the going gets tough. Remember, temporary motivations lead to temporary results.

**The Mental Aspect: Be Kind to Yourself**

Let's be real for a moment. The journey to sustainable weight loss can be rocky. There will be days when you'll feel on top of the world and others when the mirror seems like an enemy. And that's okay! Remember, you're human. Every setback is an opportunity to learn and grow. Celebrate small victories and remind yourself of your progress, not just in weight, but in strength, resilience, and self-awareness.

**Customize Your Approach**

Intermittent fasting is fantastic. But it's not a one-size-fits-all solution. Women, especially, need to tailor their fasting protocols in sync with their bodies. Some may thrive on a 16/8 method, while others might find solace in alternate-day fasting. Listen to your body, adjust, experiment, and find what works best for you.

**Focus on Nutrition, Not Just Calories**

We've all heard it: "Weight loss is a simple equation of calories in versus calories out." While there's truth to this, sustainable weight loss transcends mere math. Yes, calorie deficit is essential, but the quality of those calories matters. Prioritize whole foods, minimize processed ones, and ensure you're nourishing your body. When you focus on nutrition, you'll find you're satiated more quickly, and those cravings? They'll start to diminish.

**Holistic Wellness: Beyond the Diet**

Ladies, weight loss is not just about food. Sleep, stress, hydration, and exercise play equally pivotal roles. Embrace a holistic approach:

- **Sleep:** Ensure you're clocking in those 7-9 hours. Quality sleep aids recovery, reduces stress hormones, and curbs overeating.

- **Stress:** Chronic stress can be a weight loss saboteur. Find stress-busting activities that resonate with you, be it meditation, yoga, or simply reading a book.

- **Hydration:** Water, water everywhere, and every drop to drink! Staying hydrated boosts metabolism and aids in detoxification.

- **Exercise:** Find a routine you love. Whether it's dancing, hiking, or strength training, physical activity boosts mood, metabolism, and, of course, weight loss.

**Building a Support System**

This journey is personal, but you don't have to walk it alone. Surround yourself with positive energies. Whether it's friends, family, or a community of like-minded souls, having a support system can make all the difference. Share your highs, your lows, and everything in between. Remember, a burden shared is a burden halved.

**Realistic Goals and Non-Scale Victories**

Lastly, set realistic and achievable goals. Instead of aiming to lose 20 pounds in a month, how about starting with 5? And hey, don't be enslaved by the scale. Celebrate non-scale victories, be it clearer skin, better sleep, improved stamina, or just that joyous feeling of well-being.

**In Conclusion: Embrace the Journey**

Dear reader, sustainable weight loss is as much a journey inward as it is outward. It's about self-discovery, resilience, and tons of love and patience. As we wind up this chapter, remember, it's not about being perfect but about being persistent. So, as you step forward, know that every effort counts, every day is a new beginning, and you, yes YOU, are worth every bit of the love and care you're bestowing upon yourself. Here's to a healthier, happier, and sustainable you!

# CHAPTER 6: FASTING AND MUSCLE MAINTENANCE

## Part I: The Importance of Muscle Health

So, we've talked a lot about fasting, weight loss, and the unique facets of the female body. Now, let's pivot a bit and dive into something equally crucial, often overlooked, and super empowering – muscle health. I know, I know, you might be thinking, "But I'm not aiming to become a bodybuilder, so why should I care?" Well, let me take you on a journey that will make you view your muscles in a whole new light.

**Muscle: It's Not Just About Aesthetics**

When we think of muscles, our minds often wander to images of chiseled athletes or fitness influencers flaunting their toned biceps. But muscle health transcends aesthetic appeal. It's the bedrock of functional fitness and a crucial component of your overall well-being.

**Why Muscles Matter**

**1. Functional Strength:** Muscles enable us to perform everyday tasks with ease, be it lifting a grocery bag, playing with our kids, or getting up from a chair. A strong muscle base means better functional fitness, ensuring we can carry out our daily activities effortlessly and independently as we age.

**2. Metabolism Booster:** Muscles are metabolic powerhouses. The more muscle mass you have, the higher your resting metabolic rate. This means you burn more calories even when you're at rest. Yep, that's right, while you're binging your favorite TV show or even sleeping!

**3. Bone Health:** Muscles and bones are like the ultimate BFFs. Strong muscles lead to strong bones. Regular resistance training, which builds muscles, also increases bone density, reducing the risk of osteoporosis, especially crucial for us women.

**4. Mood Lifter:** You've heard of the "runner's high," right? Well, building and maintaining muscle can also give you a euphoric feeling. Engaging your muscles releases endorphins, those lovely feel-good hormones that combat stress and foster a sense of well-being.

**5. Chronic Disease Prevention:** Good muscle health is linked with improved insulin sensitivity, reduced inflammation, and a lowered risk of chronic diseases like type 2 diabetes and heart disease.

**Fasting: Friend or Foe to Muscles?**

Okay, so by now, you're probably nodding and thinking, "Alright, muscles are essential. But what's the deal with fasting? Will it eat away my hard-earned muscle?" That's a common concern, and honestly, a valid one.

Our body is like a finely-tuned machine. When we fast, initially, our body taps into glucose stores for energy. But as fasting continues, it needs alternate fuel. This is where fat comes into play, and our bodies begin to burn stored fat for energy. But what about muscles, you ask? Here's the cool part: our bodies are designed to preserve muscle. They don't want to use protein (from muscles) as a primary energy source. It's not efficient. Instead, the body prefers fat, especially when we're in a state called ketosis, a metabolic state where fat becomes the primary fuel.

Now, this doesn't mean muscles are entirely out of the danger zone during extended fasting. But with the right approach, you can fast and still maintain, or even build, muscle. The key lies in understanding, preparing, and taking the right measures, some of which we'll explore in the subsequent sections of this chapter.

**Incorporating Strength Training**

One of the best ways to ensure your muscles remain robust and healthy, especially if you're incorporating fasting into your lifestyle, is to engage in regular strength training. And no, this doesn't mean you need to lift super heavy weights or spend hours at the gym. Even bodyweight exercises, resistance bands, or light dumbbells can do wonders.

Strength training signals to your body that your muscles are essential and in use. This protective mechanism ensures that, even in a calorie deficit or fasting state, the body thinks twice before breaking down muscle protein for energy.

**Final Thoughts**

So, beautiful souls, muscles are more than just a pretty facade. They're a testament to our strength, both inside and out. As we venture deeper into the realm of fasting, it's crucial to give our muscles the love, respect, and attention they deserve. Because, remember, a strong woman isn't just one who can fast or eat healthily, but one who can carry her world with grace, strength, and endless vitality. And that, dear reader, is powered by the beauty of muscles.

In the next section, we'll delve deeper into the strategies to blend fasting with muscle maintenance seamlessly. Stick around; it's going to be an enlightening ride!

## Chapter 6: Fasting and Muscle Maintenance
## Part II: Protein and Fasting

So, we've journeyed through the importance of muscle health and just how pivotal it is for our overall well-being. Now, let's discuss one of the most vital elements in muscle maintenance: protein. Pair this with our ongoing topic of fasting, and we have ourselves a delicious, nutritious conversation ahead. Ready to dive in? Let's unravel the protein puzzle together!

### Understanding Protein: The Body's Building Blocks

Alright, think of your body as this magnificent structure, with every cell being a crucial brick. Now, if these cells were bricks, protein would be the cement holding them together. These are the fundamental building blocks of our body – essential for repairing cells, building new ones, and, of course, muscle maintenance and growth.

Proteins are made of smaller units called amino acids. While our body produces some amino acids, there are nine essential ones we need to get from our diet. And here's where our protein-rich foods, like meats, dairy, legumes, and grains, come into the spotlight.

### But What's Protein Got to Do with Fasting?

Great question! Here's the thing – when we fast, our body does some internal housekeeping. Old, damaged cells are cleaned out, and new ones form. Now, remember our friendly protein, the 'cement'? Yep, you guessed it – it plays a crucial role in this process.

When fasting, especially for more extended periods, it's paramount to ensure that when we do eat, our meals are rich in good-quality proteins. This ensures our muscles remain strong, and our body has the necessary amino acids for its myriad functions.

## Optimizing Protein Intake during Eating Windows

When you're incorporating intermittent fasting into your lifestyle, the timing and quality of protein intake become even more essential. Here are some tips to ensure you're nourishing your muscles appropriately:

1. **Quality Over Quantity:** Aim for high-quality protein sources, which provide all the essential amino acids. These include lean meats like chicken, turkey, and fish, dairy products like yogurt and cheese, and plant-based sources like quinoa, tofu, and lentils.

2. **Distribute Evenly:** If you're eating within an 8-hour window, for instance, try to consume protein-rich meals or snacks at the start, middle, and end of your window. This ensures a steady supply of amino acids, aiding in muscle repair and growth.

3. **Protein Shakes & Supplements:** For those especially active or struggling to get enough protein from food, protein shakes can be a boon. Opt for clean, minimal ingredient supplements, and always, always remember: supplements should not replace whole foods but should complement them.

4. **Pair with Resistance Training:** Consuming protein post-workout can aid in muscle recovery. It's like giving your muscles the tools they need to repair after a strenuous session.

## Common Misconceptions

Let's debunk a couple of myths swirling around protein and fasting, shall we?

**- "Fasting will cause muscle wastage because the body will consume all its protein."**

Not entirely accurate. As we've discussed earlier, the body prefers using fat for energy during extended fasting periods. Yes, there might be some muscle protein breakdown, but it's minimal, especially if you're ensuring adequate protein intake during your eating windows and engaging in resistance training.

- **"One should consume massive amounts of protein post-fasting to compensate."**

While protein is essential, balance is key. Consuming too much protein in one go can strain the kidneys and might not necessarily benefit muscle health. It's about consistent, evenly distributed intake.

## A Gentle Reminder for Women

For us women, especially those in their reproductive years, balancing protein intake becomes crucial, given our monthly menstrual cycle, potential for pregnancy, and unique hormonal makeup. Amino acids from proteins play a role in hormone production, so ensuring adequate intake can help balance hormonal fluctuations, which, in turn, impacts muscle maintenance.

## Final Musings

So, my dear reader, while fasting opens up a realm of benefits, it's essential to tread with knowledge and mindfulness, especially concerning protein intake. Remember, it's not about extremes but balance. Whether you're a carnivore, vegetarian, vegan, or somewhere in between, the world of protein is vast and varied. Explore, enjoy, and ensure that amidst the fasting, your muscles are singing songs of nourishment and strength.

In our next section, we'll further delve into strategies to ensure muscle health while reaping the benefits of fasting. Trust me, it's a journey worth embarking on!

## Chapter 6: Fasting and Muscle Maintenance
## Part III: Best Practices for Preserving Muscle

By now, we've explored the foundations of muscle health and how protein interacts with fasting. It's like understanding the ingredients of a recipe. Now, let's step into the kitchen and whip up the magic potion that is muscle preservation. The dance of fasting and muscle maintenance can be intricate, but oh, is it rewarding! So, put on your dancing shoes; it's time to learn the moves to keep your muscles strong and healthy during your fasting journey.

### 1. Integrate Strength Training

Strength training is the BFF your muscles have been waiting for. Not only does it build muscle, but it also signals to your body to hold onto muscle mass, especially when you're in a calorie deficit due to fasting. You don't need to become a gym rat; even body-weight exercises like squats, push-ups, and planks can work wonders. Remember, the aim is consistency, not intensity.

### 2. Protein Timing

We chatted about this a tad in our last segment, but it's worth repeating. Distribute your protein intake throughout your eating window. This ensures your muscles have a steady supply of amino acids to rebuild and repair. Post-workout protein is especially beneficial, as it's like giving your muscles the tools they need just when they need them.

### 3. Stay Hydrated

Oh, the wonders of water! Our muscles are about 75% water. Staying hydrated aids muscle function and helps in the process of protein synthesis, which is how our body uses the protein we eat. Drink up, but listen to your body – thirst is an excellent indicator.

### 4. Adequate Caloric Intake

While fasting can create a caloric deficit, which is beneficial for weight loss, it's essential not to go to extremes. Consuming too few calories can lead to muscle loss, as the body may start using amino acids for energy. Use online calculators or seek professional advice to estimate your calorie needs, and aim to meet them during your eating window.

**5. Quality Sleep**

Raise your hand if you love a good night's sleep! Sleep is the time when our bodies undergo most of their repair and recovery. A consistent sleep pattern and ensuring 7-9 hours a night can promote muscle preservation and overall health. Sweet dreams are made of these!

**6. Manage Stress**

Chronic stress can lead to muscle loss and can inhibit the body's ability to build new muscle. Activities like yoga, meditation, or even a stroll in the park can make a world of difference. Embrace them. You're not just nurturing your muscles, but your soul too.

**7. Essential Nutrients**

Protein, while a superstar, isn't the only essential nutrient. Vitamins, minerals, fats, and carbohydrates all play crucial roles. For instance, Omega-3 fatty acids can boost muscle protein synthesis and vitamin D can support muscle function. Diversify your diet to ensure you're covering all bases.

**8. Listen to Your Body**

I cannot stress this enough, darling reader. Your body communicates with you – little nudges of fatigue, the gentle hum of satisfaction after a meal, or the soreness post a workout. Listen. If you're feeling fatigued, consider adjusting your fasting window or ensuring you're meeting your nutritional needs.

**9. Consider BCAAs**

Branched-Chain Amino Acids (BCAAs) can be a good companion, especially if you work out during your fasting window. They can prevent muscle breakdown and improve workout performance. However, before jumping on the BCAA bandwagon, do your research or chat with a nutritionist to see if they align with your goals.

**10. Consistency Over Perfection**

My dear, perfection is a mirage. It's the consistent steps, the daily dance with your body's rhythms, that lead to sustainable muscle health. Whether it's your eating window, your workout routine, or your self-care rituals, it's okay to have off days. What matters is showing up, again and again.

**In Conclusion**

Muscle maintenance while fasting can seem like a tightrope walk, but with the right practices, it becomes a joyous dance. One of rhythm, balance, and harmony. Like every dance, it's unique to the dancer. And remember, it's okay to miss a step or two. The dance floor, your journey to health and wellness, will always be there, waiting for your return.

In the next chapter, we'll delve into some more advanced fasting protocols, exploring the nuances and intricacies of each. Until then, keep dancing, keep shining, and remember, you've got this!

# CHAPTER 7: MENTAL AND COGNITIVE BENEFITS

## Part I: Improved Focus and Productivity

Have you ever had one of those days when you're just **in the zone?** Time slips away as you're engrossed in a task, and before you know it, you've made a significant dent in your to-do list. That, my friend, is the magic of focus. Now, what if I told you that fasting could be a key to unlocking more of those magical days? Let's journey together into the realm of how fasting intersects with our brainpower, especially regarding focus and productivity.

**The Brain on Fasting**

To truly understand the mental benefits of fasting, it helps to picture our ancient ancestors. Think of them, roaming vast landscapes, often going without food as they hunted or gathered. Their survival depended on sharp cognitive functions during these fasting periods. Imagine trying to hunt when you can't focus on your prey! Evolutionarily speaking, it would make sense for our brains to function optimally when food was scarce. And modern science backs this up.

**Boosting Brain-Derived Neurotrophic Factor (BDNF)**

BDNF sounds like a complicated term, right? But think of it

as "brain fertilizer." It's a protein that supports brain function, mood regulation, and memory. Research has shown that fasting can increase BDNF levels, enhancing our cognitive functions and aiding focus. It's like giving your brain a little boost, readying it to tackle tasks with gusto.

## Regulation of Blood Sugar Levels

Ever felt that afternoon slump? That desire to nap right after a big meal? That's often due to a spike in blood sugar. When we fast, our blood sugar levels stabilize, leading to consistent energy levels and improved focus. No more rollercoaster highs and lows; just smooth sailing.

## The Clarity of Ketosis

A few days into a more extended fast or a ketogenic diet, our bodies enter a state called ketosis. This means we start burning stored fat for energy, producing molecules called ketones. One particular ketone, beta-hydroxybutyrate (BHB), is a super fuel for our brains. BHB has been shown to enhance brain function, clarity, and focus. It's like switching your brain from regular to premium fuel!

## Reduced Mental Clutter

You know that feeling of mental fog and clutter? It's often linked to digestion. Digesting food, especially in large amounts, requires energy. Energy that, when redirected, can leave us feeling mentally sluggish. Fasting provides our body a break from digestion, allowing more energy to be allocated to brain function. It's like decluttering your mental workspace.

## Harnessing the Power of Autophagy

Autophagy is a cellular process where our body cleans out damaged cells, making way for new, healthy ones. It's a form of self-cleaning, if you will. This process is particularly active during fasting and affects not just our body but our brain as well.

By promoting autophagy, fasting can help in clearing out neural pathways, leading to improved brain function and focus.

**Practical Tips for Maximizing Focus During Fasting**

**1. Stay Hydrated:** Even mild dehydration can impair cognition. While fasting, ensure you're drinking enough water to keep the gears of your brain well-oiled.

**2. Electrolytes are Essential:** Sometimes, an electrolyte imbalance can cause feelings of brain fog. Consider supplementing with essential minerals like magnesium, potassium, and sodium, especially during longer fasts.

**3. Break Fast Smartly:** How you break your fast can impact your post-fast cognitive function. Opt for a balanced meal with protein, healthy fats, and complex carbohydrates to maintain that focus.

**4. Mindfulness and Meditation:** Harnessing the mental benefits of fasting can be amplified with practices like mindfulness and meditation. These can train your brain to maintain focus, making the most of fasting-induced cognitive enhancements.

**5. Listen to Your Body:** Not every day will be a peak focus day, and that's okay. If you feel like your focus is waning, it might be time to reassess your fasting approach or seek guidance.

**Wrapping It Up**

Improved focus and productivity during fasting isn't just a placebo effect or a modern-day claim; it's deeply rooted in our evolutionary history. However, remember that everyone's fasting journey is unique. While many experience heightened focus, others might take time to adjust. Embrace the journey, cherish the clear-headed moments, and remember, it's a dance of tuning in and finding what works best for you.

Stay curious, dear reader, and join me as we delve even deeper into the cognitive wonders of fasting in our next segment. Every day is a chance to learn, grow, and sharpen that beautiful mind of yours.

## Chapter 7: Mental and Cognitive Benefits
## Part II: Mental Well-being and Mood Enhancements

We've journeyed through the cognitive realms of fasting, but did you know that fasting can have profound effects on our mood and overall mental well-being too? Yep, that's right. Let's dive into this enthralling topic together, shall we?

### The Mind-Body Connection

Remember the times when you've had a stomach upset and felt irritable? Or when you were overfed at a festive dinner and felt lethargic and a bit down? Our gut, often called the second brain, and our mind are intricately linked. With fasting, as we give our digestive system a break, there are cascading positive effects on our mood and mental health.

### Neurotransmitters, Our Brain's Messengers

Our brain communicates through chemicals called neurotransmitters. You might have heard of some of the big players like serotonin, often dubbed the "feel-good" neurotransmitter, or dopamine, our "reward and pleasure" messenger. Fasting influences the balance and production of these neurotransmitters, setting the stage for potential mood enhancements.

### The Serotonin Boost

You know those days when the sun is shining a little brighter, and everything feels right? That could be your brain bathing in serotonin. Research suggests that fasting can increase serotonin production. And more serotonin can translate to an uplifted mood and a feeling of well-being.

### Dopamine and Reward Sensitivity

Dopamine is like the applause our brain gives itself when we achieve something. It's that burst of joy you feel when you complete a puzzle, take a bite of your favorite dessert, or receive a compliment. Fasting has been shown to increase dopamine sensitivity, making the little joys in life feel even more rewarding.

## Reducing Oxidative Stress

Oxidative stress in the brain can lead to a dampened mood and even depressive symptoms. Fasting promotes antioxidants in the body, which combat oxidative stress, paving the way for a clearer and happier mind.

## The Calming GABA

GABA (gamma-aminobutyric acid) is a neurotransmitter that soothes the brain, preventing it from being overly active. Think of it as the calming lullaby your brain needs after a day of hustle and bustle. Fasting can increase GABA activity, promoting relaxation, reducing anxiety, and aiding in sleep.

## The Influence of Ketones

Remember our chat about ketosis in the earlier segment? Apart from fueling our brains efficiently, ketones have another trick up their sleeve: they're neuroprotective. Beta-hydroxybutyrate, the ketone we discussed, can reduce brain inflammation and promote the release of brain growth factors, enhancing mood and mental resilience.

## Practical Tips to Harness Mood Enhancements from Fasting

**1. Mindful Eating Post-Fast:** When you break your fast, pay attention to foods that nourish both body and soul. Foods rich in omega-3s (like fatty fish) and tryptophan (found in turkey, nuts, and seeds) can further boost serotonin production.

**2. Stay Active:** Physical activity complements fasting. A good walk or workout can enhance mood-improving neurotransmitter activity.

**3. Journal Your Journey:** Keeping track of your mental states during fasting can help you notice patterns and optimize your fasting regimen for mental well-being.

**4. Rest and Recover:** Make sure you're getting enough rest. Fasting can recalibrate sleep patterns, and adequate sleep is crucial for mood regulation.

**5. Stay Connected:** Sharing your fasting experiences with friends or joining fasting communities can offer social support, amplifying the positive mood effects.

**In Closing...**

Isn't it truly wondrous to think of how intricately our mental and physical states are intertwined? Through fasting, not only do we harness benefits for our body but also gifts for our mind. It's like a symphony where every component, from neurotransmitters to hormones, plays its part in creating a harmonious melody of well-being.

So, dear reader, as we continue to unravel the mysteries and marvels of fasting, remember to pause, reflect, and cherish the holistic benefits it offers. Your mind, just like your body, deserves love, care, and rejuvenation.

Join me in the next segment as we explore more about the cognitive wonders fasting brings forth. Keep shining and stay curious!

# Chapter 7: Mental and Cognitive Benefits
## Part III: The Brain-Gut Connection

You know, our bodies are truly fascinating, with countless systems intricately interwoven, each affecting the other. Have you ever had that 'gut feeling' or 'butterflies in your stomach'? There's a reason phrases like these exist in our language. Our gut and our brain are intimately connected, communicating in ways that science is just beginning to understand. Let's journey through this profound connection, shall we?

### Our Second Brain: Enter the Enteric Nervous System

Deep within our guts lies a mesh-like network of neurons, nearly as elaborate as the one in our brains, termed the Enteric Nervous System (ENS). Often dubbed our "second brain", the ENS plays a significant role in digestion and, fascinatingly, our emotional well-being. It can function independently from our central nervous system, but it often sends and receives signals to and from our brain.

### The Mighty Messengers: Neurotransmitters

You might recall our chat on neurotransmitters from the previous section. Well, hold on to your hats, because here's a startling fact: around 90% of serotonin, that "feel-good" neurotransmitter, is produced in the gut! And it doesn't stop there. The gut also produces a host of other neurotransmitters that play vital roles in our mood and cognition.

### How Fasting Affects the Brain-Gut Dialogue

When you fast, you're not just giving your digestive system a rest. You're also modifying the delicate balance of gut bacteria, which has a direct bearing on neurotransmitter production and, consequently, our mood.

**1. Balancing Gut Bacteria:** Fasting can help restore balance to our gut microbiome. A healthier balance can enhance the production of beneficial compounds, including mood-regulating neurotransmitters.

**2. Reduced Inflammation:** Fasting reduces systemic inflammation, which can have ripple effects on our gut. A less inflamed gut is better equipped to produce neurotransmitters efficiently.

**3. Improved Gut Barrier:** Periods of fasting can enhance the integrity of our gut lining, preventing harmful substances from leaching out and affecting our brain health.

**Gut Feelings and Mood**

Ever noticed how stress can mess with your digestive system, leading to upset stomachs or cravings? Or how, after certain meals, you feel lethargic and mentally foggy? It's all connected to the brain-gut dialogue.

**- Mental Stress and Gut Distress:** Chronic stress affects our gut microbiome, potentially leading to digestive issues. Conversely, an imbalanced gut can relay distress signals to the brain, exacerbating feelings of anxiety or depression.

**- Food and Mood:** The foods we consume influence our gut bacteria. For instance, a diet high in sugars and unhealthy fats can negatively impact our microbiome, potentially leading to mood swings and cognitive issues.

**Harnessing the Brain-Gut Benefits of Fasting**

**1. Mindful Eating:** When you break a fast, your gut is primed and sensitive. Consuming fiber-rich, nutrient-dense foods can nurture your gut bacteria, promoting a healthier brain-gut dialogue.

**2. Stay Hydrated:** Water aids digestion and helps maintain the mucosal lining of the intestines. Keeping hydrated during non-fasting periods supports both your gut and brain health.

**3. Probiotics and Prebiotics:** Consider integrating foods rich in probiotics (like yogurt, kefir) and prebiotics (like garlic, onions, and leeks) into your diet. These can further bolster a healthy gut microbiome, enhancing the positive effects of fasting on mood and cognition.

**4. Manage Stress:** Techniques like meditation, deep breathing exercises, and gentle physical activity can reduce stress, ensuring a harmonious brain-gut relationship.

**The Bigger Picture...**

Isn't it awe-inspiring to think of our body as this intricate web, where the state of our gut can influence the state of our mind, and vice versa? The dance between our brain and gut is a delicate one, shaped by the foods we eat, our fasting patterns, our emotions, and our environment.

So, darling reader, as you journey through the world of fasting and explore its myriad benefits, remember that by nurturing your gut, you're also cradling your mind. Every choice, every meal, every fasting window has the potential to bring harmony to this age-old dialogue between our brain and gut.

Stay tuned as we delve deeper into the cognitive wonders that fasting unravels. Keep the curiosity alive, and always trust your gut feeling!

# CHAPTER 8: AGING, LONGEVITY, AND FASTING

## Part I: Cellular Autophagy

We've embarked on quite a journey together, haven't we? From the intricate dance between our brain and gut to the power of fasting on muscle health. Today, we're going to delve into a topic that I believe holds a touch of magic. Aging. Oh, how that word conjures up so many emotions. The slow march of time, the wrinkles that trace our life's laughter and tears, the memories we cherish. But what if I told you there's a natural process, right within our cells, that can help slow the aging clock? Enter the fascinating world of cellular autophagy.

**A Journey Inside Our Cells**

Before we dive into autophagy, let's take a moment to picture our cells. Think of them as bustling little cities, with machinery and structures carrying out vital tasks. And, like any city, waste gets generated. Over time, some cellular components become damaged or obsolete. Now, if they keep accumulating, our cells become less efficient, which can lead to signs of aging and even some diseases.

But here's where it gets beautiful. Our cells have a built-in cleaning crew. This process is called autophagy.

## Autophagy: Nature's Recycling System

"Auto-" means self, and "-phagy" means eating. So, autophagy literally translates to "self-eating". But before you raise an eyebrow, let me explain. Imagine if our cities could take their old, broken-down cars and magically transform them into brand new ones. That's essentially what autophagy does on a cellular level. It breaks down damaged components and repurposes them, rejuvenating the cell.

## Why is Autophagy So Crucial?

1. **Ward off Diseases:** Inefficient or damaged cellular components can lead to inflammation and are often linked to conditions like cancer, neurodegenerative diseases, and infections. Autophagy helps reduce these risks by maintaining cellular health.

2. **Enhanced Longevity:** Some scientists believe that the activation of autophagy is one of the reasons certain organisms live longer. By continuously recycling and repairing, cells can function optimally for more extended periods.

3. **Aid in Muscle Function:** Autophagy helps in removing damaged proteins and organelles from muscle cells, ensuring they function efficiently.

## The Sparkling Link Between Fasting and Autophagy

Now, here's where our beloved fasting re-enters the story. Fasting is one of the most potent triggers for cellular autophagy. Let's understand why:

- **Nutrient Deprivation:** When we fast, our cells sense a lack of external nutrients. To compensate and sustain vital functions, they start the autophagy process to recycle components and derive the necessary nutrients internally.

- **Reduced Insulin Levels:** Fasting leads to lower insulin levels, which can stimulate autophagy. Remember our chat on insulin from the previous chapters? It's all connected, my dear reader!

**- Increase in AMPK Activation:** Fasting can activate a molecule called AMPK, a master regulator that can stimulate autophagy.

## Embracing Autophagy for Graceful Aging

While the natural aging process is beautiful and something we should embrace, the idea of aging healthfully, with vigor and vitality, is equally alluring. Here's how to tap into the powers of autophagy:

1. **Intermittent Fasting:** By now, you're no stranger to intermittent fasting. It's a brilliant way to stimulate autophagy without going on prolonged fasts.

2. **Exercise:** Physical activity, especially aerobic exercise, can also trigger autophagy. So, pair your fasting regimen with a good dose of movement!

3. **Consume Autophagy-Promoting Foods:** Green tea, coffee, turmeric, and ginger are believed to support the autophagy process. Perhaps start your day with a warm cup of green tea?

4. **Stay Hydrated:** Remember, water is essential for numerous cellular processes, including autophagy. Keep sipping throughout your non-fasting windows!

## A Glimpse Ahead...

Autophagy is a dance of renewal, a testimony to nature's genius. As we peel back the layers of the aging process and understand the role of fasting, we uncover pathways to live not just longer, but more vibrant and fulfilling lives.

Oh, the wonders that lie within us! Who knew that by simply embracing fasting, we could harness such a transformative cellular process? In our next section, we'll continue our exploration into the mysteries of longevity and the role fasting plays. Until then, keep shining, keep wondering, and remember: age is just a number when you feel alive from within!

# Chapter 8: Aging, Longevity, and Fasting
## Part II: The Role of Telomeres

I'm truly grateful for the journey we've shared so far. Through every page, every word, we're unraveling some of life's deepest mysteries, aren't we? Speaking of mysteries, have you ever wondered about the very essence of aging? What makes our cells grow old? Well, nestled within the heart of our cells, there's a secret storyteller of age called telomeres. Let's step into this wondrous world together, shall we?

### The Tale of Telomeres

Imagine for a moment your favorite pair of shoes. At the tip, there might be an aglet - that small plastic or metal sheath at the end of your shoelace. It's there to prevent the lace from unraveling. Similarly, within the intricate matrix of our DNA, there are structures called telomeres. These are like the aglets for our chromosomes, ensuring they don't deteriorate or fuse with others.

Telomeres have a challenging role. Each time a cell divides, these telomeres shorten a bit. It's a natural process but over time, as they get shorter and shorter, the cell loses its capacity to divide and becomes senescent or dies. This gradual shortening of telomeres is closely associated with aging, certain diseases, and a reduced life span. Gosh, such responsibility for something so microscopic!

### Fasting and Telomere Length

Okay, deep breath. You might be thinking, "Well, that's a bummer." But there's some magic sprinkled here. Emerging studies suggest that practices like fasting may have an impressive impact on telomere length. Let's delve into this:

**1. Reduction of Oxidative Stress:** Fasting boosts our body's antioxidant defenses. Less oxidative stress means reduced damage to our DNA and consequently, our telomeres.

**2. Enhanced Cell Repair:** When we fast, we encourage cellular repair mechanisms, including those that maintain and repair telomeres.

**3. Boosting Telomerase:** This is an enzyme that adds length to telomeres. Some research suggests fasting and caloric restriction can stimulate the activity of this vital enzyme, slowing down the shortening process and even potentially adding some length back.

### Implications of Longer Telomeres

Why should we care about these tiny structures? The implications of longer telomeres are profound:

**1. Longevity:** Longer telomeres are often seen in individuals who live exceptionally long lives. They're nature's way of granting us more turns around the sun.

**2. Reduced Risk of Chronic Diseases:** Conditions like heart diseases, diabetes, and certain cancers are linked to shorter telomeres. By maintaining their length, we might lower the risk of these ailments.

**3. Better Mental Health:** Some research hints at a connection between telomere length and mental health, including risks of conditions like depression.

**4. Enhanced Skin Health:** Skin aging is a visible sign of telomere shortening. Longer telomeres might mean a youthful skin for more extended periods!

### Nurturing Our Telomeres

Beyond fasting, what can we do to care for our telomeres? Well, darling, it's a blend of the simple joys of life and some self-discipline:

**1. Balanced Nutrition:** Antioxidant-rich foods, like berries, nuts, and green veggies, protect against oxidative stress and nurture our telomeres.

**2. Mindful Movement:** Regular exercise, be it dancing to your favorite song or a serene morning walk, can support telomere health.

**3. Meditation and Stress Reduction:** Chronic stress is a telomere's enemy. Mindfulness practices can be a haven for both your mind and your telomeres.

**4. Quality Sleep:** As you rest under a canopy of stars, your body works to repair and rejuvenate. Prioritize those restful nights.

**A Glimmer into Tomorrow**

Just imagine: nestled in every cell, telomeres silently narrate stories of our past, present, and even hint at our future. While the sands of time will always flow, it's empowering to know we can influence the pace, even if it's just a little.

Our journey doesn't end here. As we venture further, we'll uncover more mysteries of aging, longevity, and the magic fasting brings to this sacred dance of life. Hold my hand, dear reader, as we step with hope and wonder into the ever-unfolding tomorrow.

Stay radiant, stay curious, and remember: In the grand tapestry of life, every thread, no matter how tiny, weaves magic.

# Chapter 8: Aging, Longevity, and Fasting
## Part III: Anti-Aging Benefits for Women

Here we are, standing at the crossroads of time. Isn't it fascinating how the years etch stories onto our being, like an artist's canvas that deepens in detail with each passing moment? Yet, in the dance of life, many of us women sometimes wish we could slow down the tempo of aging just a smidge. And guess what? With practices like fasting, we might be holding a magical key. So, let's waltz into the realm of anti-aging and explore what it might mean for us, the nurturers, the dreamers, the warriors of time.

### Fasting: A Timeless Elixir

Fasting is an age-old practice, but did you know that beyond its spiritual and health merits, it harbors a treasure trove of anti-aging benefits for women? Here's the sparkly rundown:

**1. Skin Radiance:** Fasting can stimulate autophagy, our cells' housekeeping system. This process clears out damaged cells, making way for new ones. The result? A complexion that radiates from within, almost like you've captured the first rays of dawn.

**2. Hormonal Harmony:** As women, our dance with hormones is intricate. Fasting may optimize hormonal balance, leading to better skin health, mood stability, and even potentially easing some menopausal symptoms. Isn't it beautiful to think that by merely pausing our eating, we can serenade our hormones into harmony?

**3. Boosting Collagen Production:** Collagen is that magic protein that gives our skin its bounce and structure. With age, its production naturally declines. But guess what? Fasting could give it a gentle nudge, promoting skin elasticity and reducing those fine lines.

### Delving Deeper: Fasting's Unique Benefits for Women

Alright, wonder-woman, let's get a tad more specific. As females, our bodies and experiences with aging have nuances that are uniquely ours. Let's lovingly unwrap some of these:

**1. Bone Health:** Post-menopause, our bone density can take a hit. While more research is needed, preliminary findings hint at fasting improving bone health. Imagine, strengthening the very foundations we stand on!

**2. Mental Clarity:** Brain fog, memory lapses – sound familiar? Fasting might come to our rescue by promoting brain health, enhancing neural connections, and potentially safeguarding us against age-related cognitive decline.

**3. Emotional Balance:** Our emotional landscape is rich, intricate, and sometimes tumultuous. Some women have reported a sense of calm and emotional balance during fasting, possibly due to the stabilization of blood sugar levels.

**4. Body Composition:** As we age, maintaining a healthy body composition becomes a tad more challenging. Fasting can assist in fat loss, especially in those tricky areas, while helping preserve lean muscle mass.

**Cherishing the Journey: Tips for Women**

Alright, beauty, if you're nodding along, thinking of giving fasting a whirl, here are some tender tips, crafted just for you:

**1. Listen to Your Body:** Our bodies whisper tales of wisdom. If fasting feels right, wonderful. If it doesn't, it's okay. The journey is as unique as the twinkle in your eye.

**2. Stay Hydrated:** Water is the elixir of life. It keeps our skin plump and our bodies happy. Whether fasting or not, ensure you're sipping throughout the day.

**3. Quality Over Quantity:** When you do eat, nurture your body with wholesome foods – vibrant veggies, hearty grains, and lean proteins. Imagine you're crafting a masterpiece with every meal.

**4. Seek Support:** Connect with other women who are exploring fasting. Share stories, giggle over hiccups, and celebrate the wins. There's power in sisterhood.

**Embracing Time with Grace**

At the heart of it all, remember this: Aging is a gift, a testimony to battles won, tears shed, laughter shared, and love experienced. Fasting is merely a tool, a gentle brushstroke on the vast canvas of our lives.

Every wrinkle, every gray strand, tells a story. While we can use fasting to enhance our health and perhaps slow down the ticking clock a smidge, let's also promise to embrace each moment, each change, with grace, gratitude, and the zest for life that burns brightly within us.

In the next chapter, we'll embark on another enlightening journey. But for now, pause, breathe, and perhaps take a loving glance in the mirror. You, dear one, are time's favorite artwork, ever-evolving, ever-radiant. Keep shining.

# CHAPTER 9: FASTING AND HORMONAL BALANCE

## Part I: Balancing Estrogen and Progesterone

If there were ever a dance more intricate and delicate than that of our hormones, I'm yet to find it. Have you ever stopped to marvel at the sheer magic that our bodies perform daily? Particularly, the waltz of estrogen and progesterone – two powerful hormones that shape the experiences of those who identify as women. They influence everything from our monthly cycles to our moods. But, like any dance, sometimes our partners fall out of step. This chapter's all about guiding them back to harmony, with fasting as our compass.

**Understanding the Dance Partners: Estrogen and Progesterone**

Before diving into the rhythms and twirls, let's get to know our dancers a little better, shall we?

- **Estrogen:** Often dubbed the 'female hormone', estrogen plays an integral role in regulating the menstrual cycle, maintaining the uterine lining, and supporting secondary sexual characteristics. Beyond this, it's influential in bone health, skin hydration, and even mood stabilization.

- **Progesterone:** Consider this the calming counterpart to estrogen. Progesterone prepares the body for pregnancy and supports the uterine lining in the second half of the menstrual cycle. It has a calming effect on the body and mind and helps maintain balanced body temperature.

**When the Dance Falters: Imbalance and its Implications**

Sometimes, our dancers lose sync. This imbalance between estrogen and progesterone can lead to a myriad of symptoms:

- Irregular menstrual cycles
- PMS symptoms
- Mood swings
- Sleep disturbances
- Fertility challenges

For some, the symptoms can be subtle, a whisper of change. For others, it feels like an ongoing storm.

**Fasting: The Gentle Maestro**

Enter fasting. Imagine fasting as a gentle maestro, a conductor with the grace to guide our hormones back into their intricate dance. But how, you might wonder, can a simple act of refraining from food play such a pivotal role?

**1. Insulin Sensitivity:** Fasting can improve our body's response to insulin, a hormone deeply intertwined with our reproductive hormones. By improving insulin sensitivity, we can indirectly influence the delicate balance of estrogen and progesterone.

**2. Detoxification:** Our liver plays a starring role in metabolizing and excreting excess hormones. Fasting can support liver detoxification, ensuring hormones don't overstay their welcome.

**3. Stress Reduction:** Chronic stress can lead to progesterone depletion as the body uses it to produce the stress hormone cortisol. Fasting, particularly intermittent fasting, can reduce oxidative stress on the body, potentially preserving progesterone levels.

**Treading Carefully: What Women Should Consider**

Glorious soul, while fasting has its merits, remember this: the female body, with its ability to nurture life, has unique considerations.

- **Listening Intently:** If you're considering fasting for hormonal balance, attune yourself to your body's whispers and shouts. Some women thrive on fasting, while others might feel more fatigued. The key? Personalize the approach.

- **Shorter Fasts:** Extended fasting can be intense. For hormone balancing, shorter, more frequent fasts might be beneficial. Think along the lines of 12-16 hours rather than multiple-day fasts.

- **Nutrient Intake:** When you do break your fast, ensure you're nourishing your body with hormone-supportive foods. Think leafy greens, healthy fats, and clean proteins.

**In Harmony: Personal Stories**

Layla, a 32-year-old teacher, shared her journey with fasting. "When I started intermittent fasting, I did it for weight loss. But about two months in, I noticed something unexpected. My periods, which used to be a roller coaster of pain and mood swings, became smoother, more predictable."

Likewise, Priya, a 45-year-old entrepreneur, found solace in her fasts. "Menopause was knocking, and the symptoms were debilitating. Fasting, combined with meditation and yoga, made the transition bearable, even enlightening."

These stories are but two among countless others. They echo a sentiment that, with the right guidance and intention, fasting can indeed play a part in the symphony of our hormones.

**The Encore: Embracing the Dance**

Our hormonal landscape, with its rises and falls, mirrors the very essence of life itself. If fasting can help us find harmony, it's worth exploring. However, remember, it's not the only tool in our toolkit. Lifestyle, nutrition, sleep, and stress management are equal partners in this dance.

As we close this section, I invite you to reflect: How does your body feel today? What rhythms do you resonate with? Can fasting be your partner in this ongoing dance? Remember, dear reader, your journey is as unique as the rhythm of your heartbeat. Embrace it with love, patience, and a touch of curiosity.

In the following sections, we'll continue our exploration into the wondrous world of hormones. For now, take a deep breath, and let's cherish the dance.

## Chapter 9: Fasting and Hormonal Balance
## Part II: Thyroid Function and Fasting

Ah, the thyroid. This butterfly-shaped gland sitting at the base of our neck might be small, but let me tell you, dear reader, its impact is monumental. Have you ever felt those days when energy seems to wane, even when you've slept a solid eight hours? Or perhaps you've noticed subtle changes in your weight, without any major shifts in your diet. It's entirely possible that your thyroid might be whispering its story. Let's delve into this tale, and see how fasting fits into the narrative.

**Meet the Maestro: The Thyroid Gland**

Imagine an orchestra, with violins, cellos, trumpets, and more, each playing its part to perfection. Now, imagine the conductor, ensuring each instrument chimes in at the right time. That's your thyroid for you – the conductor of your body's metabolic orchestra.

Two primary hormones emerge from this gland:
- **T3 (Triiodothyronine):** A key hormone that regulates metabolism, energy, and growth.
- **T4 (Thyroxine):** This hormone gets converted into T3, the active form, as required by our bodies.

Together, these hormones orchestrate how our cells utilize energy. When in harmony, we feel energetic, mentally alert, and balanced. However, sometimes, this harmony goes amiss.

**Thyroid Imbalances: A Brief Overview**

- **Hyperthyroidism:** This is when the thyroid is in overdrive, producing excessive hormones. Symptoms might include anxiety, rapid heart rate, and unintentional weight loss.

- **Hypothyroidism:** The opposite of hyperthyroidism, this is a state of reduced hormone production. Fatigue, weight gain, and feelings of being perpetually cold are common indicators.

## Fasting's Serenade to the Thyroid

Now, where does fasting come into this? It's a beautiful, yet complex, serenade.

**1. Stress and the Thyroid:** Our bodies, in all their wisdom, see fasting as a form of mild stress. This might initially lead to a decrease in T3 production as the body conserves energy. For some, this is a temporary dip, and T3 levels normalize post fasting. But, and here's the catch, for others, especially with extended fasting, this might exacerbate hypothyroid symptoms. So, tread with gentle awareness.

**2. Insulin and the Thyroid:** Remember our earlier chats about insulin? Well, turns out, improving insulin sensitivity through intermittent fasting might have positive ripple effects on thyroid function. Balanced blood sugar levels can support optimal thyroid hormone production and conversion.

**3. Inflammation and Autoimmune Thyroid Conditions:** Conditions like Hashimoto's thyroiditis, an autoimmune disorder where the body attacks the thyroid, can benefit from the anti-inflammatory effects of fasting. By reducing inflammation, fasting might support thyroid function, albeit indirectly.

## A Note to the Wise: Tread Gently

My beautiful reader, if you're considering fasting and have thyroid concerns, let's pause for a moment of reflection.

**- Listen to Your Symphony:** Every body has its unique rhythm. Start with shorter fasts, monitor your energy levels, and always keep tabs on your thyroid function through regular blood tests.

**- Seek Guidance:** Collaborate with a healthcare provider who understands both fasting and thyroid health. They can be your beacon, ensuring you're supporting rather than straining your thyroid.

- **Nourish with Intention:** When breaking your fast, choose foods rich in thyroid-supporting nutrients like selenium, iodine, and zinc. Think Brazil nuts, sea vegetables, and pumpkin seeds.

## Personal Notes from the Journey

Anna, a 40-year-old artist, shared her experiences. "I have hypothyroidism and was wary about fasting. But with guidance, I tried 12-hour fasts. At first, I felt more tired, but after a week, my energy levels started to soar. Regular checks showed my thyroid function stayed stable."

On the flip side, Raj, a 35-year-old athlete, found his hyperthyroid symptoms aggravated with extended fasts. "I had to learn the hard way. Shorter fasts worked better for me."

## The Encore: Thyroid, Fasting, and You

Our thyroid, much like every part of us, sings a unique song. Fasting can be a harmonious addition to this song, but the key lies in individualized, informed choices.

Before we waltz into our next topic, let's take a moment. Close your eyes. Breathe in. Breathe out. Whisper gratitude to your thyroid, for every beat, rhythm, and note it brings to your life's symphony. Remember, in the grand orchestra of our bodies, every player, every note, matters.

Stay tuned as we delve deeper into the hormonal symphony, exploring other hormonal balances and how fasting can be a melodious guide.

# Chapter 9: Fasting and Hormonal Balance
## Part III: The Adrenal Connection

Let's talk about those tiny powerhouses sitting atop our kidneys – the adrenal glands. Ever been on a roller coaster? That rush, that thrill, that "oh my stars, what was I thinking" feeling? That's your adrenals in action. These glands might be small, but they wield significant influence, especially when fasting comes into play. Let's set out on this enlightening journey, hand in hand, exploring the dance between fasting and the adrenals.

### Adrenals: The Unsung Heroes of Stress

Have you ever thought about how we, as humans, have been built to handle stress? Whether it's missing the bus or the ever-frightening sight of your phone at 1% battery, it's our adrenals that jump into action.

These glands secrete a variety of hormones, but for today's narrative, we'll spotlight two key players:
- **Cortisol:** Often dubbed the 'stress hormone', cortisol regulates a range of processes including metabolism, reducing inflammation, and, most importantly, our natural 'fight or flight' response.
- **Aldosterone:** This unsung hero manages our salt and water balance, helping regulate blood pressure.

So, where does fasting fit into the adrenal picture?

### Fasting's Influence on the Adrenals

**1. The Initial Cortisol Surge:** When we begin our fasting journey, especially the first few times, our body sees this lack of food as a minor stressor. The adrenals respond by releasing a bit more cortisol. This isn't necessarily a bad thing! In fact, this mild spike can increase alertness and energy. Think of it as the body's way of saying, "Hey, we need to find food!" – a mechanism shaped by our ancestors' need to hunt and gather.

**2. Regulation Over Time:** As fasting becomes a more regular practice, the body gets savvier. It begins to understand there's no immediate threat of starvation. For many, cortisol levels may stabilize over time with consistent fasting routines. However, it's important to note, everyone's dance is unique.

**3. Impact on Blood Pressure:** Remember our friend, Aldosterone? Fasting can lead to decreased sodium levels in the blood. The adrenal glands may release aldosterone to balance this, drawing sodium back into the bloodstream. This is why some fasting guides recommend a pinch of salt in your water – it's all about harmony!

**Walking the Tightrope: Balance is Key**

While the adrenal response to fasting can be beneficial, we must approach this dance with a sense of balance. Chronic stress – whether from life's many curveballs or excessive, improperly managed fasting – can overburden the adrenals.

**- Adrenal Fatigue:** Imagine constantly asking a friend for favors, day in and day out. Eventually, they might feel drained, right? Similarly, if our adrenals are continuously pumping out cortisol due to constant stress and insufficient recovery, they can get weary, leading to a state often referred to as 'adrenal fatigue'. Symptoms might include chronic fatigue, mood swings, and weight gain.

**Fasting with Adrenal Awareness**

If you have adrenal concerns or if life's stresses are weighing heavily on your shoulders, let's tread the fasting path with tender care.

**- Shorter is Sweeter:** Instead of long fasts, consider shorter, more manageable intervals. This can offer the benefits without overtaxing the adrenals.

**- Nourishment is Key:** When breaking a fast, indulge in

nutrient-rich foods. Think foods high in vitamin C like bell peppers and strawberries, which are fantastic for adrenal support.

- **Mindfulness Matters:** Pair fasting with stress-reducing practices like meditation or deep breathing. This holistic approach ensures you're supporting your adrenals and not just demanding from them.

**Your Symphony, Your Pace**

Let's hear from Lisa, a 28-year-old teacher, "I dived headfirst into fasting, excited by its promises. But with the demands of my job and personal stresses, I found myself drained. I learned the importance of balance. Now, I fast, but I also meditate and prioritize self-care."

Your body, your symphony. Every note, every pause, every crescendo – it's uniquely yours. The adrenals, just like any other instrument, play a pivotal role. Fasting can be a beautiful tune in this composition, but always remember to play it at a pace that resonates with your being.

As we close this chapter on the adrenal connection, take a moment. Place a hand on your heart, breathe deeply, and send a wave of gratitude coursing through your body, especially to those tiny glands juggling so much. In this vast concert of life, they play their part, note by note, beat by beat, ensuring the music never stops.

# CHAPTER 10: FASTING DURING DIFFERENT LIFE PHASES

## Part I: Puberty and Adolescence

Now, let's venture into an ever-evolving and delicate period of life—puberty and adolescence. If you're a teenager reading this, or perhaps a parent, guardian, or educator seeking to understand, know that this chapter is crafted with utmost empathy and care.

**The Symphony of Change: Puberty Explained**

Imagine the body as an orchestra. Until puberty, the instruments played relatively simple tunes. But then, a conductor—let's call it 'hormones'—decides it's time for a richer, more complex composition.

Puberty, this vibrant mélange of physical, emotional, and cognitive changes, is spurred by these hormonal shifts. This phase transforms children into young adults, equipping them with the ability to reproduce and bestowing them with secondary sexual characteristics. It's nature's way of saying, "Hey, you're transitioning, and it's going to be one heck of a ride!"

**Fasting During this Delicate Phase**

**1. The Energy Question:** Teen years are bustling! There's school, sports, extracurriculars, and that whirlwind of social dynamics. These activities demand energy. Fasting, especially without proper guidance, might reduce the vital fuel adolescents need to power through their day.

**2. The Growth Factor:** Adolescents are in their prime growth phase. Bones elongate, muscles develop, organs grow— it's like a 24/7 construction site. Caloric and nutritional intake is crucial. While fasting has its merits, it's essential to ensure it doesn't compromise the necessary nutrients during this period.

**3. Emotional and Cognitive Impact:** The teenage brain is like wet cement—still setting and shaping. Emotional highs and lows are typical, thanks to those hormonal shifts. Fasting can further affect mood, concentration, and cognitive functions. Being attentive to these changes is crucial.

**Considering Fasting? Points to Ponder**

Are you an adolescent, toying with the idea of fasting? Or perhaps a concerned adult? Let's walk through some critical checkpoints:

- **Reasoning Matters:** Ask the all-important 'why'? Is it religious, health-focused, or perhaps influenced by peer or societal pressure? Understanding the motivation helps in tailoring a safe and effective approach.

- **Nutritional Safety Net:** If fasting is embarked upon, ensure there's a safety net of nutrients. It's not just about the absence of food but what you consume before and after. Nutrient-dense meals, rich in protein, healthy fats, and vitamins, are pivotal.

- **Hydration, Hydration, Hydration:** The young body is bustling with metabolic processes, all requiring water. Even during fasts, keeping hydrated is non-negotiable.

- **Listen to Your Body:** It might sound clichéd, but attuning to your body's signals is paramount. Feeling dizzy, overly fatigued, or emotionally drained? It's a sign. Pause and reassess.

**The Educator's and Parent's Role**

Dear adults, your guidance, understanding, and support can make all the difference. Here are some suggestions:

- **Open Conversations:** Create a safe space for dialogue. If your adolescent wishes to fast, understand their reasons, and discuss the potential challenges and benefits.

- **Be Observant:** Watch for signs of extreme fatigue, mood swings, or any other drastic changes. It's essential to differentiate between typical teenage behavior and potential fasting side effects.

- **Educate on Balance:** While it's crucial to respect their choices, it's equally vital to emphasize balance. Guide them on how they can integrate fasting without compromising their overall well-being.

**Final Notes: A Letter to the Young Reader**

Puberty and adolescence are intricate, beautiful, sometimes overwhelming, but always transformative. It's a journey of self-discovery, of understanding the deep caverns of your mind and the ever-changing landscape of your body.

If fasting beckons you, remember: your worth isn't measured by the hours you abstain from food. Listen to your body, cherish its signals, and nourish it. You're in a phase where every nutrient plays a pivotal role in sculpting the future you.

And to the guardians of these young souls, tread with understanding and empathy. They look up to you, even if they don't always show it. Your guidance is their compass in this intricate phase.

In our next segment, we'll explore fasting during adulthood. Until then, embrace every beat of your heart, every breath, every change. Because, my dear reader, every phase is a melody in the vast symphony of life.

Stay tuned, and let's continue this enlightening journey.

## Chapter 10: Fasting During Different Life Phases
## Part II: Pregnancy and Postpartum

Here we are, stepping into one of the most magical, intense, and transformative phases in a person's life: pregnancy and the postpartum period. These moments are packed with profound emotions, physical transformations, and endless questions. For many, one of those questions is about fasting. Let's navigate this together, hand in hand.

### Pregnancy: The Miracle of Life

Every beat of your heart now echoes with another's. With every inhale, you breathe not just for yourself but for the tiny life blooming inside of you. Pregnancy is a miracle, a dance of biology and love. Yet, it's also a time of heightened responsibility, where every decision can impact the little one growing inside.

### Fasting During Pregnancy: Delving into the Why's and How's

**1. Nutritional Needs:** During pregnancy, your body demands a richer tapestry of nutrients. From folic acid to iron, calcium to vitamin D, these aren't just fancy names on a prenatal vitamin bottle; they're the building blocks of your baby's development. Fasting can sometimes make it challenging to meet these increased needs.

**2. Blood Sugar Levels:** Maintaining stable blood sugar levels is vital. Sudden drops, which can happen during extended fasts, might not only leave you feeling faint but can also impact the steady flow of nutrients to your baby.

**3. Hydration:** Amniotic fluid, increased blood volume, breast tissue expansion—your body is like a sponge during pregnancy, needing more water than ever. Extended fasting can risk dehydration, which isn't something you'd want to flirt with during this time.

## Postpartum: Welcoming a New Dawn

The storm and beauty of childbirth have passed, and you're now cradling your world in your arms. Yet, the postpartum period can be a whirlwind. From sleepless nights to navigating breastfeeding, your body and mind are still very much in flux.

### Fasting in the Postpartum Phase

**1. Breastfeeding and Nutritional Demands:** If you're breastfeeding, know that it's a calorie-intensive process. Your body might need an extra 300-500 calories daily to produce milk. Fasting might challenge this increased caloric need, potentially affecting milk supply.

**2. Physical Recovery:** Childbirth, be it a natural delivery or a C-section, takes a toll. Your body is in repair mode, and depriving it of nutrients during extended fasts might not be the wisest choice.

**3. Emotional Well-being:** Hormonal shifts, sleep deprivation, and the sheer weight of new responsibilities can make the postpartum phase emotionally intense. Fasting can sometimes amplify mood swings or feelings of fatigue.

### Considering Fasting? Here's What to Keep in Mind

- **Consult a Healthcare Professional:** This isn't just standard advice—it's essential. Every pregnancy and postpartum journey is unique, and your doctor or midwife can offer tailored guidance.

- **Shorter, Gentler Fasts:** If you're keen on fasting, consider shorter intervals. Maybe a 12-hour overnight fast, ensuring you're hydrating and breaking the fast with nutrient-rich foods.

- **Listen, Listen, Listen:** Tune into your body's signals. Feeling exhausted, dizzy, or overly emotional? It might be time to reconsider your fasting decision.

**A Note to Partners and Support Systems**

Your role is irreplaceable. Be the pillar of understanding, ensuring the new mother has all she needs, from a glass of water to emotional support. If she's considering fasting, be a part of the conversation, learn together, and make informed decisions as a team.

**Dear Blossoming Mother**

You're incredible. Every stretch mark, every sleepless night, every sacrifice speaks volumes of your strength and love. As you navigate the choice of fasting during this phase, remember: you're doing the best you can. Trust yourself, lean on your support system, and always prioritize what feels right for you and your baby.

The journey of life has many phases, each with its challenges and beauty. As we inch closer to understanding fasting's role in each of these phases, our next segment will touch upon menopause and the golden years.

# Chapter 10: Fasting During Different Life Phases
## Part III: Menopause and Beyond

The tapestry of life is woven with threads of change. It's the transformations, both subtle and monumental, that frame our existence. And as women, the transition into menopause is one of those landmark shifts—a complex intersection of biology, emotion, and spirituality. Like every phase, it has its challenges, its beauties, its stories. And within these stories, many women seek to understand the place of fasting.

Let's embark on this journey together, understanding the dance between fasting and this unique phase of womanhood.

### Understanding Menopause: A Symphony of Changes

Before we delve into fasting, it's crucial to understand what menopause is all about. Gone are the monthly cycles, and in their place, a symphony of hormonal changes ensues. Ovulation ceases, estrogen and progesterone levels decrease, and the body finds its new rhythm. For some, it's a gentle transition, while for others, it can be like a rollercoaster of hot flashes, mood fluctuations, and sleep disturbances.

### Fasting During Menopause: The Prospects and Caveats

**1. Weight Management:** One of the most common narratives during menopause is the shift in weight distribution and metabolism. For many, fasting offers a potential solution for weight management. The calorie restriction and potential metabolic benefits can aid in combating the weight gain that some experience during this phase.

**2. Hormonal Balance:** The decrease in estrogen levels during menopause can lead to various symptoms. While fasting has shown potential in regulating insulin and stress hormones, its direct impact on estrogen and progesterone remains a topic of exploration. However, some women find that intermittent fasting helps in achieving a semblance of balance.

**3. Bone Health:** A significant concern during menopause is bone density, as declining estrogen levels can lead to osteoporosis. It's essential to understand that while fasting has myriad benefits, prolonged fasting without adequate nutrient intake can be detrimental to bone health.

**4. Mood and Mental Well-being:** The hormonal shifts can sometimes play games with one's mood. Interestingly, some women find clarity and improved mental wellness during fasting periods. This might be linked to the ketone production in the body during extended fasts, which some studies suggest can be neuroprotective.

**The Golden Years: Aging Gracefully with Fasting**

Post-menopause, the journey doesn't end. Instead, it metamorphoses into the golden years—a phase of introspection, liberation, and often, rediscovery. How does fasting fit in here?

**1. Cellular Health:** As we touched upon in earlier chapters, fasting can induce cellular autophagy—a natural cleansing mechanism. This can be particularly beneficial in the later years, promoting cellular health and combating the wear and tear that comes with age.

**2. Cognitive Function:** Aging sometimes brings with it the shadows of cognitive decline. The potential neuroprotective benefits of fasting, primarily through ketone production, can be a beacon of hope for maintaining cognitive sharpness.

**3. Digestive Wellness:** With age, the digestive system might not be as sprightly as it once was. Fasting offers a break, a pause, allowing the system to rest and rejuvenate.

**Navigating Fasting During These Phases: A Compass of Consideration**

- **Personalized Approach:** No two bodies are the same. Your experience with menopause and the years that follow is unique.

Thus, your fasting journey should be tailored to you. Listen to your body—it speaks, often in whispers, sometimes in shouts.

- **Nutrient-Rich Diet:** Especially crucial during these years is a diet rich in calcium, vitamin D, and other essential nutrients. If you choose to fast, ensure that your eating windows prioritize these nutrients.

- **Consultation is Key:** Seek the guidance of healthcare professionals. Discuss your intentions, understand potential risks, and make informed decisions.

- **Hydration:** Especially in the face of hot flashes and potential dehydration, sipping water throughout the day becomes paramount.

## A Note to the Soul Reading This

You're a testament to resilience, grace, and the profound depth of womanhood. Menopause and the years that follow aren't just about aging or hormonal shifts—it's about embracing change, growing, and continuing to bloom. As you contemplate fasting, remember it's just one of the many tools in your vast toolbox. Cherish yourself, embrace every phase, and know that you are, and will always be, a wonder.

Onward, dear reader, our journey of discovery and understanding continues. With each chapter, we unravel a bit more, and there's still so much left to explore. Onwards, with love and light.

# CHAPTER 11: SOCIAL AND LIFESTYLE ASPECTS

## Part I: Navigating Social Events

The air is filled with music, there's the clinking of glasses, laughter, and the tantalizing aroma of food wafts through. Ah, social events! Whether it's a wedding, a weekend brunch, a birthday bash, or a simple dinner date, our lives are sprinkled with these moments of togetherness. They're not just about the food or the drinks; they're about connection, celebration, and shared memories. But what happens when your chosen fasting window clashes with these events? Suddenly, the joyous occasion might be clouded by stress or anxiety. Let's chat about this, dear friend. How can you stay true to your fasting goals and still relish the heartbeats of life?

**Understanding the Challenge**

First and foremost, it's essential to acknowledge the challenge. Fasting is not merely a physical act; it's intertwined with our emotions, societal norms, and, often, deep-rooted habits. Social events, particularly those centered around food, can become a minefield of temptations and peer pressure. "Oh, come on, just one bite!" or "Are you on a diet AGAIN?" might be common phrases you hear. Remember, it's okay to feel conflicted, and it's okay to seek a balance.

**Tips to Sail Smoothly Through Social Waters**

**1. Flexibility is Your Friend:** One of the beauties of intermittent fasting is its flexibility. If you know you have a dinner event, consider shifting your eating window for that day. It's not about being rigid; it's about finding what suits you best in the current circumstance.

**2. Communicate, Communicate, Communicate:** Talk to your friends or family about your fasting journey. When they understand your reasons and goals, they're more likely to support you. It's also a chance to dispel myths or concerns they might have.

**3. Have a Snack Beforehand:** If the event falls just outside your eating window, consider having a light, healthy snack before. This way, you won't be ravenously hungry, and you'll be less likely to overindulge.

**4. Hydration Station:** Keep a glass of water or herbal tea in hand. It not only keeps you hydrated but also gives you something to sip on, which can be especially helpful if you're feeling out of place without food.

**5. Focus on the Non-Food Aspects:** Engage in conversations, dance, laugh, play games. Immerse yourself in the joy of being with your loved ones. Food is just one component of these gatherings.

**6. Plan Ahead with the Host:** If you're comfortable, speak to the host ahead of time. They might offer alternatives or at least be aware of your choices. And who knows? There might be others on a similar journey.

**7. Mindful Eating:** If you do choose to eat, make your choices mindfully. Savor each bite, relish the flavors, and appreciate the nourishment. This also helps in preventing overeating.

**8. Don't Let a Misstep Derail You:** So you broke your fast a bit early, or you indulged more than you intended. That's okay. Remember, every meal, every moment is a new beginning. Don't be too hard on yourself.

**Dealing with Peer Pressure**

This can be one of the trickiest parts. Society has deeply ingrained beliefs about eating, celebrations, and togetherness. A few strategies to manage this include:

- **Polite but Firm:** If someone insists you eat, thank them for their concern, explain briefly, and redirect the conversation.

- **Find Allies:** You'd be surprised at how many people are curious about or even practicing fasting. They can be your companions in navigating the event.

- **Focus on the Positive:** Instead of explaining why you're not eating, maybe share the benefits you've experienced from fasting, turning the narrative around.

**In Conclusion: Celebrate Life, Your Way**

The journey you've undertaken with fasting is deeply personal. It's about listening to your body, understanding your rhythms, and seeking well-being. Social events are a part of the beautiful tapestry of life, moments of joy and togetherness. By planning ahead, communicating openly, and practicing flexibility, you can navigate these occasions with grace and joy.

As we continue this journey together, remember that fasting isn't just about when you eat; it's about crafting a lifestyle that resonates with you. So, here's to celebrating life, with all its flavors and nuances, while staying true to our paths. Cheers!

# Chapter 11: Social and Lifestyle Aspects
# Part II: Combining Fasting and Fitness

Fitness, much like fasting, is a journey of self-discovery, discipline, and pushing the boundaries of what we believe is possible. As we embark on a fasting journey, many of us wonder, "How will this choice intersect with my fitness goals?" To those of you scratching your heads, mulling over your gym schedules, and rethinking that morning jog, let's dive deep together and unravel this conundrum.

## Understanding the Interplay

At first glance, fasting and fitness might appear at odds. After all, conventional wisdom dictates that we need fuel before a workout and nourishment post-exercise for recovery. But the human body, my dear friend, is a marvel of adaptability. It's capable of so much more than we give it credit for. So, while there's an adjustment period, combining fasting and fitness is not only possible but can also be incredibly rewarding.

## The Benefits of Fasting Workouts

**1. Enhanced Fat Burn:** When you exercise in a fasted state, your glycogen (stored sugar) levels are lower. This pushes your body to tap into fat stores for energy, making your workouts more efficient at burning fat.

**2. Increased Growth Hormone Production:** Fasting is known to stimulate the release of growth hormone, which aids muscle growth and recovery. When combined with exercise, this effect can be amplified.

**3. Improved Insulin Sensitivity:** Both fasting and exercise independently improve insulin sensitivity. Together, they can supercharge this effect, helping your body utilize glucose more effectively.

**4. Mental Clarity:** Many people report heightened focus and clarity during fasted workouts, possibly due to the ketones produced during fasting, which are a potent brain fuel.

**Finding Your Rhythm**

Now, not all workouts are created equal, and neither are all fasting windows. The key lies in experimentation and listening to your body.

**1. Low-Intensity Workouts:** Activities like walking, yoga, or light aerobic exercises can usually be performed at any time during the fasting window without any issues. They're gentle on the system and can even be soothing.

**2. High-Intensity Workouts:** These might require more strategizing. Some find it best to engage in high-intensity interval training (HIIT) or weightlifting towards the end of their fasting period, followed by a nutrient-dense meal. Others prefer to fuel up with a meal and then hit the gym a couple of hours later.

**3. Hydration is Key:** Whether you're sipping on water, herbal teas, or electrolyte-infused beverages, staying hydrated during workouts, especially when fasting, is crucial. This aids performance and recovery.

**4. Listen to Your Body:** This can't be stressed enough. While many thrive on fasted workouts, if you feel lightheaded, excessively fatigued, or just "off," it might be a sign to adjust your routine or eat something pre-workout.

**Nutrition and Recovery**

Combining fasting and fitness doesn't mean neglecting nutrition. It's about optimizing it.

**1. Post-Workout Nutrition:** If your workout coincides with your eating window, focus on consuming protein to aid muscle recovery and healthy carbs to replenish glycogen stores. A smoothie with protein powder, almond milk, and a banana, for instance, can be a great post-workout treat.

**2. Stay Mindful of Calories:** While fasting can help regulate appetite, combining it with rigorous exercise might increase hunger levels. It's essential to eat enough to support your activity without overindulging.

**3. Micronutrients Matter:** Minerals like magnesium, potassium, and sodium can be lost through sweat. Ensure you're replenishing these, especially if you're working out during fasting hours.

## Social Aspect of Fitness and Fasting

Often, our fitness routines have a social component—be it a gym buddy, a group class, or a community run. Combining this with fasting can raise eyebrows or concerns from well-meaning friends.

**1. Open Conversations:** Much like navigating social events, it's beneficial to communicate with your fitness pals about your fasting journey. Sharing research, personal experiences, and the reasons behind your choices can foster understanding.

**2. Find a Fasting Workout Buddy:** Having someone on a similar journey can be both motivating and comforting. You can share tips, experiences, and perhaps even recipes for that delicious post-workout smoothie.

## In Conclusion: Crafting Your Unique Dance

Combining fasting and fitness is like choreographing a dance—sometimes gentle, sometimes dynamic, but always uniquely yours. Remember, it's not about rigid rules but about fluidity, understanding, and most importantly, listening to the melodies of your body.

As you lace up those sneakers or roll out that yoga mat, know that you're not just building muscles or burning calories, but you're also crafting a symphony of well-being, one beat, one breath at a time. Let's keep dancing, shall we?

# Chapter 11: Social and Lifestyle Aspects
## Part III: Fitting Fasting into a Busy Lifestyle

Let's be real for a moment. Our modern lives are a whirlwind of tasks, responsibilities, and commitments. Meetings overlap with soccer games. Work deadlines clash with family dinners. Self-care routines? They sometimes feel like luxuries we can't afford. Into this bustling mix, you're thinking of adding fasting? Well, believe it or not, this ancient practice might be the modern solution to balance you've been seeking.

### Embracing the Flexibility of Fasting

One of the most beautiful aspects of fasting is its innate flexibility. It's not about a rigid schedule set in stone, but about crafting a rhythm that dances in tune with your life. No two days are identical, and neither should your fasting approach be.

**1. Flexible Windows:** While consistency can be beneficial, if a 16-hour fast doesn't fit into your Tuesday because of a breakfast meeting, adjust. Maybe that day, you opt for a 14-hour window, or perhaps you switch to a different kind of fasting method, like the 5:2 approach.

**2. Weekday vs. Weekend Fasting:** Some people find it easier to fast during the working week when they're swamped with tasks and then relax their schedule over the weekend. Remember, it's about finding what feels sustainable and harmonious for you.

### Preparation is Half the Battle Won

Having a plan can make a world of difference. Just as you might schedule meetings or block off time for certain tasks, think of fasting as another appointment—a sacred one—with yourself.

**1. Meal Prep:** If you know you'll be breaking your fast during a particularly busy period, prepare your meal in advance. This ensures you refuel with nutritious options instead of reaching for the nearest convenience food.

**2. Fasting Apps:** Many mobile applications can help you track your fasting windows, send you reminders, and even offer tips and motivation during those hunger pang moments.

**3. Stay Hydrated:** Always have a water bottle on hand. This not only helps stave off hunger but ensures you're well-hydrated, especially crucial during busy days that can lead to inadvertent neglect of basic needs.

## Merging Mindfulness and Multitasking

While the buzzword 'multitasking' often gets a bad rap, when combined with mindfulness, it can be a potent ally in your fasting journey amidst a hectic schedule.

**1. Mindful Eating:** Even if you have just 15 minutes for a meal, make it count. Put away distractions, savor each bite, and truly appreciate the nourishment you're providing your body. It might be the most grounding part of your day.

**2. Mindful Breaks:** Got 5 minutes between tasks? Instead of mindlessly scrolling on your phone, take a few deep breaths, stretch, or simply close your eyes. These moments, peppered throughout your day, can make the fasting journey smoother and more connected.

## Navigating Social and Professional Commitments

A jam-packed calendar might mean breakfast events, lunch meetings, or dinner dates. While these can pose challenges, they're also opportunities to reimagine how fasting fits into your social life.

**1. Communicate:** Let people know about your fasting journey. You'd be surprised how many might be curious, supportive, or even share their own experiences.

**2. Adjust Your Window:** If you have a dinner date, consider shifting your eating window to accommodate it. Fasting is about flexibility, not rigidity.

**3. Order Smartly:** If you're at a social event during your fasting window, opt for non-caloric beverages. Herbal teas, sparkling water with a slice of lemon, or even plain water can be your best friends.

## A Little Kindness Goes a Long Way

Lastly, amidst the hustle and bustle, always prioritize kindness —towards yourself. Some days, the fasting window might be shorter; other days, you might miss it altogether. And that's okay.

**1. Acknowledge Effort:** Celebrate the days you successfully incorporate fasting into your schedule. And on days you don't? Recognize the effort, learn, and move forward.

**2. Seek Support:** Connect with a community, be it online forums, local groups, or friends on a similar journey. Sharing experiences, tips, and challenges can offer both motivation and a sense of camaraderie.

## Wrapping it Up

As the sun sets on another bustling day, and you find a quiet moment to reflect, let's remember this: Fasting, in its essence, is a pause. A pause from eating, yes, but also an invitation to pause from the incessant pace of life, to reconnect with our bodies, our needs, and our inner selves. In the modern symphony of responsibilities and deadlines, think of fasting as your solo—a moment to shine, to be truly present, and to serenade your soul.

# CHAPTER 12: FASTING AND GUT HEALTH

## Part I: Understanding the Gut Microbiome

As you delve deeper into the world of fasting, you might have come across the term "gut microbiome" more than once. You might be wondering, "What's this all about?" or "Why should I care about these tiny organisms living inside me?" Here's the kicker: This community of microorganisms residing in your gut has profound effects on your health, mood, and, yes, even how you think! Let's embark on this journey of understanding our gut's bustling ecosystem and its fascinating interplay with fasting.

**The Fascinating World Inside You**

Imagine a bustling city, teeming with life, activity, and diversity. Now, scale that down a few hundred times, and you have your gut microbiome. This vast community, mostly comprising bacteria but also viruses, fungi, and other microorganisms, calls your gastrointestinal system home.

**1. Diversity is Key:** Just like any city thrives on the variety of its inhabitants, the gut's health is directly linked to the diversity of its microbial residents. A rich and diverse gut microbiome is often associated with better overall health.

**2. Symbiotic Relationship:** These microorganisms aren't freeloaders. They help break down complex foods, produce essential vitamins, and even play a role in regulating our immune system.

**The Gut-Brain Connection**

Yes, you read that right. Your gut and brain are in cahoots. They're constantly chatting, sending signals back and forth. Ever had a 'gut feeling'? It's not just a saying; it's biology.

**1. Mood Modulators:** Some strains of bacteria in the gut produce neurotransmitters, like serotonin—the feel-good hormone. A healthy gut can mean a happier you.

**2. Stress Responders:** Ever noticed tummy troubles during stressful times? Stress impacts gut health, and in turn, an imbalanced gut can heighten stress responses.

**How Diet Influences the Gut**

Your gut microbiome is a reflection of your dietary habits. Just as you crave a variety of foods, so do these tiny organisms.

**1. Fiber Fanatics:** Beneficial bacteria thrive on dietary fiber found in fruits, vegetables, and whole grains. A diet rich in these helps maintain a balanced microbiome.

**2. Sugar Slump:** On the contrary, diets high in sugars and processed foods can lead to an overgrowth of less beneficial bacteria. Remember, it's all about balance.

**Enter Fasting: A Respite for Your Gut?**

Now, where does fasting fit into this intricate dance of the gut? Let's break it down:

**1. Rest and Repair:** Fasting gives your digestive system a break. This pause allows the gut lining, which might be damaged due to various factors, a chance to repair.

**2. Microbial Reset:** Just like you sometimes need a reset, so does your gut. Fasting can help in rebalancing the microbial community, favoring the growth of beneficial bacteria.

**3. Boosting Beneficial Compounds:** Fasting can lead to an increase in the production of certain compounds, like short-chain fatty acids, which have anti-inflammatory properties and are beneficial for gut health.

**Personalizing Your Fasting Approach**

Everyone's gut is unique—like a fingerprint. This means the way your gut responds to fasting might differ from your friend's.

**1. Listen to Your Gut:** If you experience discomfort, like bloating or constipation, during fasting, it might be a sign to tweak your approach or consult with a health professional.

**2. Hydration is Key:** Water aids digestion and ensures the smooth functioning of the gut. During fasting, make sure you're adequately hydrated.

**3. Breaking the Fast:** What you eat post-fast is crucial. Consider foods that are easy on the digestion and rich in fibers, like soups, broths, or smoothies.

**Conclusion**

Our understanding of the gut microbiome is like an unfolding novel, with new chapters of discoveries being written regularly. What's clear, however, is the profound connection between our health and these unseen residents of our body.

Fasting, in many ways, offers a bridge—a bridge to better gut health, a bridge to understanding our bodies better, and perhaps, a bridge to a more harmonious existence with the millions of microorganisms we share our lives with.

Remember, dear reader, as you navigate the winding paths of fasting, sometimes the answers you seek aren't just in the vast expanse outside but in the incredible universe within. Here's to celebrating the mysteries, wonders, and potential of our gut microbiome!

# Chapter 12: Fasting and Gut Health
## Part II: Fasting's Effect on Gut Flora

Hey again, intrepid explorer of health and well-being! We've just journeyed through the bustling city within – our gut microbiome. Now, we're taking a deeper dive to understand how fasting affects this intricate community. Think of it as understanding how a long weekend might affect the dynamics and mood of a buzzing metropolitan. Ready? Let's journey onward!

### Fasting: A Time of Feast or Famine for Gut Bacteria?

Imagine you've decided to clean up your house, and suddenly, there's this unexpected clarity and space. Similarly, fasting provides our gut a metaphorical "spring cleaning". Let's see what happens to our gut residents during this process.

**1. Shift in Power Dynamics:** When we fast, we deprive gut bacteria of their regular food source. This might sound a little cruel, but it can lead to a decline in some bacteria, especially those that thrive on our regular diet. This gives other, often beneficial, bacteria an opportunity to flourish and take the lead.

**2. The Rise of Resilient Bacteria:** Some gut bacteria are hardy little beings. They can withstand longer periods without food, and fasting brings these resilient ones to the forefront. These bacteria, interestingly, are often the kinds that produce substances beneficial for our gut lining and overall health.

### Butyrate Producers: The Unsung Heroes

Butyrate – no, it's not a new diet fad, but it's worth its weight in gold when it comes to our gut.

**1. Who are they?** Certain gut bacteria produce butyrate as a by-product. Butyrate is a short-chain fatty acid that plays a crucial role in maintaining the health of our intestinal walls.

**2. Fasting's Gift:** Fasting appears to increase the abundance of these butyrate-producing bacteria. Why's this a good thing? Well, butyrate is like a superfood for the cells of our colon. It reduces inflammation, strengthens the gut barrier, and even has anti-cancer properties!

**Supporting the Mucus Layer**

**1. The Mighty Mucus:** Our gut has a protective mucus layer, which serves as a barrier and home for many bacteria. Certain bacteria feed on this mucus layer when there's no food around.

**2. What Fasting Does:** During fasting, there's an increase in these mucus-feeding bacteria. While this might sound alarming, it's a natural adaptive response. As they feed on the mucus, they produce compounds beneficial for the gut. However, it's a delicate balance. Prolonged fasting without replenishing might thin out this protective layer too much.

**Enhancing Gut Immunity**

Our gut is not just a digestion chamber; it's a fortress, the front line of defense against harmful pathogens.

**1. Guarding the Gates:** Within our gut lies a vast network of immune cells, ready to combat any harmful invaders. Fasting helps in the regeneration of these cells, essentially bolstering the defenses of our fortress.

**2. Friend or Foe?** With fasting, our gut becomes better at distinguishing between friendly bacteria and potential pathogens. This means a reduced risk of unnecessary inflammation and better cooperation with beneficial bacteria.

**Post-Fasting: The Reintroduction Phase**

Imagine coming home after a vacation. It takes a while to settle back, right? Similarly, when we reintroduce food after fasting, our gut flora goes through a phase of adjustment.

**1. Diversity Spike:** Introducing varied and fiber-rich foods post-fasting can lead to a bloom in bacterial diversity. This is a plus point, as diversity is a marker of a healthy gut.

**2. Listening to Feedback:** Your gut will communicate with you. If certain foods cause discomfort post-fasting, it might be a sign that your gut flora is adjusting, or that you need to reintroduce such foods more gradually.

**Practical Tips: Nourishing Your Gut Post-Fast**

**1. Go Slow:** Think of breaking your fast as waking up gently from a deep slumber. Introduce foods gradually, starting with easy-to-digest options.

**2. Fiber is Your Friend:** Foods rich in fiber, like fruits, vegetables, and whole grains, encourage the growth of beneficial bacteria.

**3. Stay Hydrated:** Water aids in digestion and helps maintain the health and balance of the gut flora.

**4. Monitor and Adjust:** Keep an eye on how different foods make you feel. Adjust based on your body's feedback.

**In Conclusion**

As we wind up this chapter, remember that our gut flora isn't just a passive community. It's dynamic, responsive, and plays a pivotal role in our overall health. While fasting has its benefits, it's essential to approach it with awareness, listening to the feedback our bodies provide.

Every fast is a journey, a dance of intricacies between us and the trillions of microorganisms residing within. When done right, it's a dance that can lead to harmony, health, and a deeper understanding of the wondrous ecosystem that is our body.

Till our next chapter, may your gut flora bloom and your health blossom! Remember, you're not just eating (or fasting) for one; you're doing it for trillions!

## Chapter 12: Fasting and Gut Health
## Part III: Fasting for Digestive Issues

Let's set the stage. You've had a long day. You're looking forward to sinking into your favorite armchair with a good book (perhaps this one!). But suddenly, your tummy starts its own symphony - a cacophony of rumbles, gurgles, and maybe even a sharp pang or two. It's your gut reminding you it exists, and not in the best of ways. Sound familiar?

If you've ever battled digestive issues, you know they're not just "in your stomach". They can affect your mood, energy, and overall well-being. In this chapter, we'll unravel how fasting might be a potent tool in your arsenal against digestive troubles. Journey with me through the intricate maze of our digestive system!

### The Digestive Break: Why Fasting Can Help

Imagine working tirelessly, day in and day out, without a break. That's precisely what our digestive system does. Every bite, sip, snack – it's all processed by this tireless machinery. Fasting, in essence, gives your digestive system a well-deserved vacation.

**1. Rest and Repair:** When we fast, our stomach and intestines get to pause, not having to break down and absorb food. This pause can help the gut lining heal and regenerate.

**2. Reducing Inflammation:** Chronic inflammation can be a root cause of many digestive disorders. Fasting has been shown to decrease markers of inflammation, giving our gut a breather and a chance to recover.

### Fasting for Specific Issues

**1. Irritable Bowel Syndrome (IBS):** IBS is like that unpredictable friend – you never know what mood they'll be in! Symptoms can range from diarrhea to constipation, bloating, and pain. Fasting can help reset the gut, reduce inflammation, and regulate bowel movements. However, it's essential to reintroduce foods slowly and note any triggers.

**2. Acid Reflux and GERD:** These conditions result from stomach acid creeping into the esophagus. Not pleasant, right? Fasting, by reducing the amount of acid production, can provide relief. However, when breaking your fast, opt for alkaline and non-spicy foods.

**3. Bloating and Gas:** Sometimes, our gut bacteria have a feast, producing gas as a byproduct, leading to that uncomfortable bloated feeling. A short fast can help reset this, but remember, it's crucial to be mindful of the foods you reintroduce.

## Cautions and Considerations

While fasting can be a powerful ally, it's not a one-size-fits-all solution. Consider the following:

**1. Not a Magic Bullet:** Fasting can aid in relief, but it's essential to address underlying dietary and lifestyle habits. Relying solely on fasting without making other changes can be like putting a band-aid on a wound that needs stitches.

**2. Listening to Your Body:** This can't be stressed enough. If you feel severe discomfort while fasting, it might be a sign that your body needs something different. It's okay to break a fast if it doesn't feel right.

**3. Seek Professional Advice:** If you suffer from severe digestive issues, please consult with a healthcare professional before embarking on a fasting journey. They can provide guidance tailored to your situation.

## Hydration and Electrolytes: The Silent Guardians

When fasting, especially for those with digestive troubles:

**1. Stay Hydrated:** Drink plenty of water. Dehydration can exacerbate digestive discomfort.

**2. Mind the Electrolytes:** Fasting can lead to a drop in essential minerals. Consider incorporating a pinch of pink Himalayan salt in your water or drinking bone broth to keep electrolytes in balance.

## Mindfulness: The Digestive Anchor

Remember, our gut isn't just affected by what we eat, but also how we eat.

**1. Slow and Steady:** When you break your fast, eat slowly. Savor each bite. This not only aids in digestion but also helps you recognize when you're full.

**2. Chew, Chew, and Chew:** Digestion begins in the mouth. Properly chewing food makes it easier for the stomach and intestines to process.

## In Conclusion

Our gut, this incredible maze within, plays a pivotal role in our overall well-being. While the idea of fasting can seem daunting, especially if you're grappling with digestive issues, it offers a beacon of hope for many. But always remember, you're the captain of your ship. Listen to your body, seek guidance when needed, and embark on this journey with knowledge and mindfulness.

Here's to a happier, healthier gut, and a more vibrant you. Digestive peace is not just a dream – with the right tools, it's within grasp. Onward, dear reader, to more chapters and more revelations!

# CHAPTER 13: POTENTIAL SIDE EFFECTS AND SOLUTIONS

## Part I: Common Concerns and Remedies

Hello again, dear reader! As we've ventured deep into the world of fasting, I've aimed to share its myriad of benefits with you. But like any good story, there are two sides to consider. So, let's dive into some of the common concerns and hiccups people encounter when fasting, and most importantly, some gentle remedies to help you along the way. It's all part of the journey, after all.

**1. Feeling Faint or Lightheaded**

It's a peculiar feeling – that slight dizziness when you stand up or perhaps an unsteady sensation when you're just moving around.

**Why It Happens:** A drop in blood sugar or blood pressure can often lead to these feelings.

**The Remedy:** Drink plenty of water. Dehydration can exacerbate lightheadedness. If it continues, consider breaking your fast with a light, balanced snack, or consult a healthcare professional.

## 2. Headaches

Oh, the nagging pain of a headache. It's as if someone's doing a little tap dance on your temples, right?

**Why It Happens:** Reduced caffeine intake, dehydration, or the body adjusting to burning fat instead of glucose can be the culprits.

**The Remedy:** Start by sipping some water. If you regularly drink caffeine, consider tapering down before starting a fast. Gentle stretches or a short walk in fresh air can also alleviate tension.

## 3. Difficulty Sleeping

You're in bed, staring at the ceiling, wondering about the mysteries of the universe while the rest of the world snoozes away.

**Why It Happens:** Increased adrenaline levels during fasting can lead to insomnia.

**The Remedy:** Try winding down with a routine: a warm bath, some calming tea (caffeine-free), or meditation can work wonders. Ensure your sleeping environment is cool, dark, and comfortable.

## 4. Digestive Discomfort

Whether it's constipation or its mischievous cousin diarrhea, digestive hiccups can be, well… a bit of a bother.

**Why It Happens:** A sudden change in eating patterns can throw our digestive system off balance.

**The Remedy:** Stay hydrated. For constipation, consider a warm cup of herbal tea. When breaking your fast, reintroduce foods gently and monitor how your body responds.

## 5. Bad Breath

You're having a chat, and suddenly you're more conscious of your breath than the words you're saying.

**Why It Happens:** When your body switches to burning fat, it produces ketones—one of which, acetone, is released in the breath.

**The Remedy:** Regularly brushing your teeth and drinking water can help. Sugar-free chewing gum or mints can also be temporary saviors—just be cautious about the artificial sweeteners in them.

**6. Mood Fluctuations**

One moment you're on top of the world, and the next, you're a bit irritable. It's like an emotional roller coaster.

**Why It Happens:** The body's adjustment to new energy sources, changes in blood sugar, and hormonal shifts can lead to mood changes.

**The Remedy:** Take some deep breaths and give yourself grace. Recognize this as a part of the adjustment process. Engaging in calming activities or taking short breaks can be beneficial.

**7. Muscle Cramps**

Suddenly, a wild muscle cramp appears! It's not very effective at making you feel good.

**Why It Happens:** Electrolyte imbalances, especially reduced sodium and magnesium, can lead to cramps.

**The Remedy:** Sipping on water with a pinch of pink Himalayan salt can help. Also, consider eating foods rich in magnesium, like leafy greens and nuts, when you're not fasting.

**Facing Concerns Head-On**

When embarking on a fasting journey, it's natural to have hesitations. And that's okay. Remember, you're not alone. Many before you have navigated these waters and come out feeling renewed and rejuvenated. With every potential side effect, there's a solution, a remedy—a way to make things better.

**Final Thoughts**

As we wrap up this part, I want to leave you with a thought: every journey has its bumps, its unexpected turns, and maybe even a pit stop or two. But it's those very challenges that make the destination all the more rewarding.

Stay hydrated, stay informed, and most importantly, stay kind to yourself. You've got this, dear reader. Onward we go, exploring, understanding, and growing.

## Chapter 13: Potential Side Effects and Solutions
## Part II: Recognizing When to Break the Fast

Ever been on a long road trip and thought, "Maybe it's time to pull over for a bit"? Fasting can sometimes feel like that journey. While the road stretches ahead with promise, it's essential to know when to pause, refuel, and maybe even enjoy the view for a while. Let's chat about understanding those signs and signals that tell you, "Hey, it might be time to break this fast."

### 1. Intense Hunger

Not the usual "Hmm, I could eat" kind of hunger, but the gut-deep, almost painful hunger that's hard to ignore.

**What's Happening:** Initial hunger pangs are common as you start fasting, but if they persist or become unbearable, it's a clear sign your body is asking for sustenance.

**Listening to Your Body:** Intuition can be a powerful guide. When the hunger feels intense and distracting, it's okay to break your fast. Nourish yourself with a balanced meal, and remember, every fasting journey is unique.

### 2. Severe Fatigue

While mild tiredness can be part and parcel of the fasting process, persistent fatigue or lethargy isn't.

**What's Happening:** Your body might be running very low on its energy reserves, indicating that it's time to refuel.

**Listening to Your Body:** Rest when you can, and if the fatigue doesn't lift, consider ending your fast. Listen to that inner voice saying, "I need a pick-me-up," and opt for nutritious, energy-boosting foods.

### 3. Mental Fog or Confusion

Having trouble focusing? Words jumbling up or tasks seeming

way harder than usual?

**What's Happening:** This could be due to a drop in blood sugar or a sign that the body needs energy.

**Listening to Your Body:** If your cognitive functions feel hampered, it's crucial to break the fast, especially if you're in a setting that requires concentration, like driving or working.

### 4. Overwhelming Mood Fluctuations

It's natural to have mood swings from time to time, but if you're feeling unusually emotional or irritable, it's a signal worth noting.

**What's Happening:** Hormonal fluctuations and changes in blood sugar levels can impact mood.

**Listening to Your Body:** Self-awareness is key. Recognize heightened emotions as a potential sign, and consider breaking the fast with mood-stabilizing foods like complex carbs and protein.

### 5. Persistent Digestive Discomfort

More severe than the occasional tummy rumble or digestive hiccup, persistent discomfort can indicate it's time to eat.

**What's Happening:** Your digestive system might be signaling it's ready for some action!

**Listening to Your Body:** Introduce light, easily digestible foods first. Hydration is also essential—sip on warm water or herbal tea.

### 6. Heart Palpitations

Feeling your heart race or skip beats can be unnerving, and it's vital not to ignore these signals.

**What's Happening:** Electrolyte imbalances or dehydration can sometimes lead to palpitations.

**Listening to Your Body:** Always play it safe when it comes to the heart. Break your fast and hydrate. If palpitations persist, seek medical attention immediately.

### Being Kind to Yourself

Reading these signs might make fasting sound daunting, but remember, it's about tuning in and really listening to what your body has to say. Each of us is beautifully unique—what feels right for one person might be different for another. And that's okay.

There's no failure in breaking a fast. Every time you choose to fast, you're giving yourself a fresh experience, a new insight into your body's rhythms and needs. It's like dancing—you learn the steps, find the rhythm, and sometimes, you step on a toe or two. But the dance goes on!

### The Beauty in Flexibility

Fasting is as much an art as it is a science. While the science gives us guidelines, the art lies in the adaptability, the gentle curves and detours we take based on our feelings and needs.

If you find yourself thinking, "Is it time to break the fast?", reflect on it. There's wisdom in your intuition, in those gentle nudges and louder shouts from within.

### Final Musings

Dear reader, as we drift towards the end of this chapter, remember that fasting is a journey filled with highs and lows, with moments of clarity and challenges. But every step, every moment, is rich with insight and learning.

Hold onto your kindness and patience, for these are your guiding stars. And as you navigate the intricate tapestry of fasting, remember—you're not alone. We're on this journey together, learning, evolving, and growing with every sunset and sunrise.

Until our next heart-to-heart, be well, be gentle, and most of all, be you.

# Chapter 13: Potential Side Effects and Solutions
# Part III: The Role of Hydration

Diving into another chapter together, I want you to visualize something for a moment. Picture an oasis in a desert—a sparkling pool surrounded by palm trees. Imagine how crucial that water is for the life that thrives in that harsh environment. In many ways, our bodies are similar. In the midst of the intense practice of fasting, hydration becomes our oasis, our lifeline.

Let's uncover the magic and absolute necessity of hydration, especially when we're exploring the journey of fasting.

## 1. Why Water is Your Best Friend During Fasting

You've probably heard this a million times, but it's worth repeating: our bodies are predominantly water. About 60% of our bodies, to be precise. So, when we decide to withhold food during a fast, the role of water becomes even more significant.

**The Cleanser:** When fasting, our bodies go into a mode of detoxification. Water aids in flushing out toxins, supporting our kidneys in the natural detox process.

**The Energizer:** Even though you're not consuming calories, water can be a source of energy. How? By helping in the transportation of nutrients and supporting cellular functions. Think of it as your secret weapon against fasting fatigue.

## 2. Electrolytes: The Unsung Heroes

Apart from pure water, there's another hydration-related topic we need to dance with—electrolytes. These are minerals that carry an electric charge and play a crucial role in maintaining many of our bodies' essential functions.

**Balancing Act:** Electrolytes like potassium, sodium, and magnesium help maintain the balance of fluids in and out of our cells, tissues, and organs.

**Symphony of Signals:** Our nerve reactions and muscle function (yes, that includes your heart!) rely on the perfect balance of these electrolytes. Ever had a muscle cramp during fasting? That's your body's SOS for more electrolytes.

### 3. Hydrating Right: It's Not Just About Quantity

Drinking water is fantastic, but chugging gallons without listening to your body isn't the way to go.

**Sip, Don't Gulp:** Slow, consistent hydration throughout the day can be more beneficial than flooding your system all at once. Listen to your body's cues and hydrate accordingly.

**Natural Electrolyte Boosters:** Before you rush to the store for a sports drink (which can often be filled with sugar and artificial ingredients), consider natural sources. Coconut water, a pinch of sea salt in your drinking water, or even a splash of lemon can help replenish lost minerals.

### 4. Recognizing Dehydration

While we're on this journey, it's important to recognize when we're straying off the hydration path:

**Thirst is Late:** By the time you feel thirsty, you might already be mildly dehydrated. Keep a bottle nearby as a visual reminder to drink up.

**The Color Test:** Paying a visit to the loo? Check the color. Dark yellow? Time to hydrate. Aim for a light, pale straw hue.

**Other Clues:** Dry skin, fatigue, headache, or dizziness can all be whispers (or shouts) from your body asking for more hydration.

### 5. Overhydration: Yes, It's a Thing

In our enthusiasm, sometimes we can go overboard. Drinking excessive water can dilute our blood, leading to an imbalance in our electrolyte levels, a condition called hyponatremia.

**Balancing is Key:** It's about harmony. Don't force water down, but also don't neglect it. Aim for balance and intuition-led hydration.

### 6. Infused Waters: Making Hydration Fun!

If you're missing the joy of flavors during fasting, infused waters might be your savior. A slice of cucumber, a sprig of mint, or a few berries can make your hydration journey refreshing and delightful. Plus, you get some added nutrients seeping into your drink!

### Deep Dive Conclusion

Diving back up from our hydration exploration, it's evident how intertwined water is with our well-being, especially when navigating the fasting seas. As with everything in life and fasting, balance and attunement to one's body are the compass and map.

Remember, lovely reader, you are the best advocate for your health. While the world offers advice and knowledge, the true wisdom rests within you. Feel the rhythm of your needs, and let it guide your hydration choices.

As we wrap up, picture that oasis again. Let it be a reminder of the calm, nourishing, and refreshing role water plays in our journey. Until our next chat, raise a glass of water to your health and well-being! Cheers!

# CHAPTER 14: INTEGRATING NUTRITION WITH FASTING

## Part I: Macronutrient Balancing

You've made it through quite a journey with fasting, and now, we're about to sprinkle in some nutritional magic. Remember, fasting isn't just about when you eat, but also what you eat. The orchestra of our body thrives when each instrument—protein, fats, and carbohydrates—plays in harmony. So, let's delve deep into the world of macronutrients and explore how we can balance them with fasting.

### 1. What are Macronutrients, Anyway?

Before we start our balancing act, let's get clear on what macronutrients are. In the vast world of nutrition, macronutrients (or "macros" for short) are the three main categories of nutrients that provide us with energy:

**Proteins:** The building blocks of life, aiding in tissue repair, muscle building, and hormone production. Think of proteins as the bricks and mortar of your body's house.

**Fats:** No, they're not the enemy! Fats are essential for brain health, hormone production, and nutrient absorption. They're the insulation in the walls of our house.

**Carbohydrates:** Our body's primary energy source, carbs are like the fuel that keeps our house's furnace burning.

## 2. Fasting and Protein: Building and Repairing

When you fast, the body undergoes various processes, including cellular repair. This is where protein plays a starring role.

**Preserving Muscle Mass:** While fasting, it's vital to ensure you're consuming enough protein during your eating windows to maintain muscle mass.
**Sources Matter:** Opt for clean protein sources such as lean meats, fish, legumes, and tofu. Imagine you're giving your body the finest building materials to work with.

## 3. Fats: Nourishing Every Cell

There's been so much debate about fats over the years. But let's set the record straight—they're absolutely essential, especially when fasting.

**Satiety is Key:** Healthy fats keep you fuller for longer, making your fasting period smoother.
**Omega-3s and Brain Health:** Including sources like flaxseeds, walnuts, and fatty fish can boost your mood and cognitive function.
**Cooking with Healthy Fats:** Using olive oil, coconut oil, or ghee can elevate your dishes and nourish your body.

## 4. Carbohydrates: Timing and Selection

Ah, carbs—so loved, yet so misunderstood. With fasting, it's not just about how many carbs you eat, but when and which types you choose.

**Glycemic Index (GI):** This is a measure of how quickly a food can raise blood sugar. When breaking a fast, lean toward low-GI foods like quinoa, lentils, or sweet potatoes to avoid sudden spikes.

**Carbs Post-Workout:** If you're combining fasting with fitness, consider consuming carbs post-workout to replenish glycogen stores.

**Fruits and Veggies:** Remember, not all carbs are bread and pasta! Fruits and vegetables are carb sources too and come packed with essential vitamins, minerals, and fiber.

## 5. Personalizing Your Macro Ratio

There's a lot of chatter out there about the "perfect" macronutrient ratio—40:30:30, high carb, low fat, high protein, and so on. But here's the deal: your body is uniquely yours.

**Listen to Your Body:** Start with a balanced approach and then adjust based on how you feel. Do you have more energy? Are you satiated between meals? Use these cues to tweak your intake.

**Consider Your Goals:** If you're aiming to build muscle, you might lean into more protein. If you're into endurance sports, maybe carbs take center stage.

**Seek Professional Guidance:** If you're unsure, consider consulting a nutritionist or dietitian. They can offer personalized advice and adjustments.

## 6. Macro Balance: A Fluid Dance

Just like everything in life, the balance of macronutrients isn't a rigid structure. It's a fluid dance, changing with your life stages, activities, and health goals.

**Adapt and Adjust:** Maybe during winter, you crave more hearty, fatty foods, while summer sees you leaning into fruits and salads. That's okay! Embrace the ebb and flow.

**Your Body, Your Rules:** At the end of the day, macronutrient balance should serve **you** and not the other way around. Enjoy the journey of discovery and adaptation.

## Dive-Deep Wrap-Up

As we wind down our chat on macronutrients, I hope you're

feeling empowered. Combining the practice of fasting with mindful nutrition is like creating a masterpiece—a symphony of well-being, harmony, and vitality.

Remember that nourishing your body is a profound act of self-love. As you navigate this journey, let intuition and self-awareness be your guiding stars. After all, the ultimate goal isn't just about numbers or ratios, but celebrating the vibrant, dynamic being that is you.

# Chapter 14: Integrating Nutrition with Fasting
## Part II: Micronutrient Importance

While we've just ventured through the broad strokes of macronutrients, let's now dive into the intricate world of micronutrients. Think of macronutrients as the broad brushstrokes on a canvas, while micronutrients are the delicate details that bring the masterpiece to life. Let's explore these small yet mighty heroes of our nutrition and see how they play their part during fasting.

### 1. Micronutrients: A Quick Overview

Micronutrients, often referred to as vitamins and minerals, are required in trace amounts but are **vitally important** to our health. These are the nutrients that don't necessarily provide energy like macros do but are instrumental for countless bodily functions.

**Vitamins:** Organic compounds crucial for our body's physiological processes. Examples include Vitamin C, a powerhouse antioxidant, and Vitamin D, the sunshine vitamin.
**Minerals:** Inorganic nutrients that play a pivotal role in many of our body's systems. Think calcium for bones or magnesium for muscle function.

### 2. Fasting and Micronutrient Absorption

When you fast, your digestive system gets a break. This could potentially increase the efficiency of nutrient absorption when you eat.

**Empty Canvas:** After fasting, your digestive tract is like a fresh canvas, potentially more receptive to the vibrant colors (or nutrients) you introduce.
**Quality over Quantity:** Especially during fasting, focus on nutrient-dense foods to ensure you're absorbing a wide spectrum of vitamins and minerals in limited meals.

### 3. Key Micronutrients to Monitor

While all micronutrients are essential, a few need special mention, especially when you're integrating fasting into your lifestyle:

**Iron:** Crucial for energy and transporting oxygen in our blood. Especially for menstruating individuals, ensuring an adequate intake of iron-rich foods like leafy greens or lean meats is pivotal.
**Magnesium:** This mineral is a star player in muscle function, energy production, and even mood regulation. Nuts, seeds, and whole grains are your go-to sources.
**Potassium:** Think heart health and fluid balance. Fruits like bananas and oranges, as well as veggies like spinach and potatoes, are rich in this vital mineral.
**B Vitamins:** A complex of several vitamins, they're vital for energy, brain function, and creating red blood cells. Whole grains, eggs, and legumes are great sources.

### 4. Micronutrients & Energy During Fasting

When fasting, it's common to sometimes feel a tad sluggish. Ensuring you're getting a full spectrum of vitamins and minerals can help regulate energy levels.

**Natural Energy Boost:** While your morning coffee might give you a jolt of energy, micronutrients sustain it. Vitamins like B12 play a key role in energy production.
**Brain Power:** Omega-3 fatty acids, often discussed in the realm of fats, are crucial for brain health and can help maintain cognitive function during fasting periods.

### 5. How to Maximize Micronutrient Intake

While fasting narrows down our eating window, it doesn't mean we need to skimp on nutrient quality. Here are some tips:

**Rainbow Plate:** Aim to eat a variety of colors on your plate. Each color often represents different vitamins and minerals. So, bring on the colorful veggies and fruits!

**Whole Foods:** Processed foods often strip away essential nutrients. Embrace whole, unprocessed, or minimally processed foods for maximum benefit.

**Hydration Helps:** While not a micronutrient, water assists in the absorption of several vitamins and minerals. Keep sipping throughout the day!

## 6. Supplements: Do I Need Them?

The world of supplements can be both enticing and confusing. But do you really need them?

**Listen to Your Body:** If you're feeling consistently drained, it might be worth checking your micronutrient levels. A simple blood test can guide you.

**Professional Guidance:** Before diving into supplements, consult a healthcare professional. They can provide insights tailored to your unique needs.

**Food First:** Always aim to get your micronutrients from food first. Supplements can complement but shouldn't replace a balanced diet.

## 7. Respecting Our Body's Symphony

It's fascinating, isn't it? Our bodies are like grand orchestras, with every instrument (or nutrient) playing its unique part. When one is off-key, it affects the entire ensemble.

Remember, dear reader, that our bodies, with their intricate needs and signals, are deeply wise. As you integrate fasting into your life, remember to honor the small, subtle whispers of your body. Whether it's craving a juicy orange (hello, Vitamin C!) or a handful of nuts (thanks, magnesium!), your body knows.

Cherish these cues, embrace the journey, and remember: you're not just eating food, you're absorbing life, energy, and vitality. Each micronutrient, though minute, is a drop in the vast ocean of your well-being.

With each bite, you paint your canvas. Make it vibrant, make it colorful, make it **you**.

# Chapter 14: Integrating Nutrition with Fasting
## Part III: Supplements and Fasting

While we've marveled at the intricate dance of macronutrients and the quiet, powerful force of micronutrients, there's another area of nutrition that beckons our attention: supplements. In our quest to perfect fasting and ensure we're nourishing our bodies, the question arises – where do supplements fit into this tapestry?

### 1. Setting the Stage: What Are Supplements?

First off, let's clear the air. Supplements are exactly what they sound like – a supplement to our diet, not a replacement. They offer concentrated doses of certain nutrients, be it vitamins, minerals, or other beneficial compounds.

**Remember, in the beautiful opera of our body's functions, supplements are the understudies, stepping in when the lead actor (our nutrition from food) might be falling a bit short.**

### 2. Why Consider Supplements While Fasting?

When you're fasting, especially for extended periods, there might be days when you don't quite get every nutrient your body craves. Here's where supplements can step in:

**Filling Nutrient Gaps:** Even with the most meticulously planned meals, there might be days you miss out on certain nutrients.

**Special Diets:** For those on restrictive diets – vegan, keto, or others – some essential nutrients might be challenging to obtain from food alone.

**Boosting Health Goals:** Whether it's improving immunity, increasing bone density, or enhancing skin health, targeted supplements can give you that extra nudge.

### 3. The Go-To Supplements During Fasting

Ah, the vast universe of supplements! Let's shine a spotlight on a few that might be particularly beneficial when integrating fasting into your lifestyle:

**Multivitamins:** Think of these as an insurance policy. They can cover a broad spectrum of vitamins and minerals, ensuring you don't miss out on essential nutrients.
**Vitamin D:** Especially if you're living in places with limited sunshine or are mostly indoors, a Vitamin D supplement can be a boon for bone health and mood.
**Omega-3 Fatty Acids:** Fantastic for heart and brain health, these fats are often found in fish oil or algae-based supplements, especially useful for those who don't consume fish.
**Electrolytes:** Extended fasts can sometimes deplete our body's electrolyte balance. An electrolyte supplement can assist in hydration and muscle function.

## 4. Timing: When to Take Your Supplements?

Supplements during fasting can be a bit tricky. After all, you're aiming to maintain that "fasted" state. Here's a roadmap:

**Water-Soluble Vitamins:** These, like Vitamin C or the B vitamins, can typically be taken during your fasting window without breaking the fast.
**Fat-Soluble Vitamins & Oils:** Vitamins like A, D, E, and K, or supplements like fish oil, are best taken with meals to enhance absorption.
**Minerals:** If you're taking mineral supplements, like magnesium or calcium, it's often best with meals to prevent any potential stomach discomfort.

## 5. The Possible Sidekicks: Digestive Enzymes and Probiotics

When fasting, our digestive systems get a breather. But when it's time to eat, some folks might benefit from a little digestive support.

**Digestive Enzymes:** These can assist in breaking down foods, ensuring maximum nutrient absorption, especially if you have a sensitive tummy.

**Probiotics:** Boosting gut health, these beneficial bacteria can support digestion and even boost immunity. A happy gut is often a happy you!

## 6. Supplements: Not One-Size-Fits-All

It's essential to remember that supplements are deeply personal. What works wonders for your friend might not be the best for you.

**Always Consult a Healthcare Professional:** They can provide insights tailored to your unique needs and health goals.

**Less Can Be More:** It's tempting to jump into the supplement bandwagon, but sometimes simplicity is key. Start slow, monitor how you feel, and adjust accordingly.

## 7. Listening to Your Body's Whispers

Throughout our fasting journey, there's one resounding theme: listening. Listen to the quiet nudges, the subtle signals that your body sends you. Feel a bit off? Maybe you need a boost of a particular nutrient.

And remember, while supplements can offer a safety net or a boost, they aren't magic pills. The real magic? It's in the wholesome, colorful, and diverse foods you eat, the water you sip, the air you breathe, and the love and care you shower upon yourself.

In this tapestry of health and well-being, supplements are threads, weaving in and out, providing strength where needed. But the real art? It's you, dear reader. It's in every choice you make, every bite you take, and every moment you dedicate to nurturing yourself.

Till our next chat, keep shining, keep listening, and keep

exploring the wondrous world of nutrition and fasting. Here's to a healthier, happier you.

# CHAPTER 15: EMOTIONAL AND PSYCHOLOGICAL ASPECTS

## Part I: Relationship with Food

Diving deep into fasting, you've probably realized that our relationship with food isn't just about the physical nourishment it provides. It's tangled with emotions, memories, and habits that have been brewing over years. Let's talk about that intricate dance between our minds, hearts, and our plates.

### 1. Food: A Tapestry of Emotions

Have you ever reached for a tub of ice cream after a break-up? Or nostalgically remembered your grandmother's cookies on a gloomy day? Food isn't just sustenance; it's tied with memories, comfort, celebration, and sometimes, even consolation. Our emotions can, quite literally, shape our appetites.

### 2. The Comfort Food Phenomenon

Ah, the allure of mac n' cheese, warm pies, or a bowl of rich, creamy soup. Comfort foods. They're not just tasty; they're emotionally fulfilling. But why?

**Memory Lane:** Often, these foods are tied to warm, cherished memories—cozy family dinners, festive holidays, or loving moments.

**Brain Chemistry:** Foods, especially those rich in carbs and fats, can boost the production of serotonin—a feel-good neurotransmitter.

### 3. The Cycle of Emotional Eating

While leaning on food for comfort occasionally is a universal experience, it can become a recurring pattern for some. This is where emotional eating enters.

**Stress? Eat. Guilt? Eat Again:** Stress or emotional upheaval can lead to binge eating. But once the initial comfort wears off, it's replaced by guilt, leading to another round of stress eating. Recognizing this cycle is the first step to breaking it.

### 4. Fasting: An Opportunity to Reflect

Fasting can become a mirror, reflecting our relationship with food. Without the regularity of meals, you might:

**Confront Cravings:** Is it hunger? Or is it a craving intertwined with emotions? Fasting provides a pause, a moment to ask, "What am I truly hungry for?"
**Break Habits:** Maybe you're used to a chocolate bar every afternoon. Fasting can help you discern if it's a true need or just a deeply ingrained habit.

### 5. Setting Boundaries: It's Okay!

As you deepen your fasting practice, you'll sometimes face internal pressures. "Should I really break my fast now? But it's only been X hours!" Here, it's crucial to remember that your emotional well-being is paramount.

**Listen to Your Emotions:** If fasting is causing undue stress or making you obsessively think about food, it's okay to recalibrate. Your emotional health is just as crucial as physical health.
**Seek Balance:** While discipline is a part of fasting, rigidity isn't.

Finding a balance where fasting enhances your life rather than controlling it is the sweet spot.

### 6. Rediscovering Food Joy

Amidst the schedules, timings, and plans, don't forget the simple joy of savoring food—the burst of flavors, the textures, the colors.

**Mindful Eating:** When you break your fast, try eating without distractions. Savor each bite, be present, and truly relish the experience.
**Gratitude:** Before you eat, take a moment to express gratitude—for the food, the hands that prepared it, and the earth that nurtured it.

### 7. When to Seek Help

It's essential to remember that while fasting can offer insights into your relationship with food, it's not a remedy for deep-seated food-related challenges.

**Recognize the Signs:** Constant anxiety around food, extreme guilt after eating, or using fasting as punishment can be signs that you need to seek professional help.
**Reach Out:** If you feel your relationship with food is impacting your mental well-being, consult a therapist or counselor specializing in eating disorders or food-related challenges.

**In Conclusion...**

Your journey with fasting is more than just about when you eat; it's an exploration of your relationship with food, your emotions, and, essentially, yourself. Like any relationship, there'll be ups and downs, moments of clarity, and moments of doubt. But every step, every insight, every challenge is a part of this wondrous journey.

So, dear reader, as you sip on your water or your tea, take a moment to appreciate this intricate relationship. And remember, while food nourishes the body, understanding, kindness, and self-love nourish the soul.

Sending you a virtual hug and wishing you a journey filled with self-discoveries and heartfelt moments.

# Chapter 15: Emotional and Psychological Aspects
## Part II: Overcoming Fear of Hunger

Oh, hunger. The rumbling tummy, the slight lightheadedness, that gnawing feeling that seems to shout, "Feed me now!" Many of us have grown up in environments where food is abundant, and the slightest pang of hunger sends us darting to the pantry. But, my dear reader, today we're embarking on a heart-to-heart journey. We're addressing the elephant in the room (or should I say, the hunger in the stomach?): the fear of hunger.

### 1. Unraveling the Fear

Hunger isn't just a physical sensation; it's deeply intertwined with our emotions and psychology. From the comforting memory of a childhood snack to the societal notion that hunger equates to deprivation, our relationship with this feeling is complex.

The first step? Acknowledge that your fear of hunger is valid. It's rooted in evolution (our ancestors needed to eat when they could), cultural beliefs, and personal experiences.

### 2. Understanding Hunger vs. Appetite

Let's demystify this duo:

**Hunger:** It's our body's physiological signal indicating the need for food. Think of it as your fuel gauge notifying you that it's time for a refill.
**Appetite:** This is the desire to eat, often tied to emotions, surroundings, or specific cravings. Ever had a full meal and still fancied a slice of chocolate cake? That's appetite talking.

Distinguishing between these two can be enlightening. The next time your stomach growls, ask yourself, "Is this genuine hunger, or am I just in the mood for something tasty?"

### 3. Embrace the Benefits

Hunger, especially during fasting, isn't a foe; it's a sign that your body is transitioning into a state where it starts to burn stored fat for energy. It means you're stepping into a zone of numerous health benefits – autophagy (cell repair), enhanced brain function, and improved insulin sensitivity, to name a few.

## 4. Mindful Check-ins

When hunger strikes, instead of reacting impulsively, pause. Take a deep breath. Check-in with yourself:

"How am I feeling?"
"Is this hunger linked to an emotion?"
"What does my body truly need right now?"

You'll often find that it's not food you're seeking but comfort, distraction, or even hydration.

## 5. Redefine Your Relationship with Food

We eat for various reasons - joy, comfort, celebration, or out of sheer habit. By recognizing and understanding these patterns, you can start to redefine your relationship with food:

**Emotional Eating:** If you're eating because of stress, sadness, or boredom, consider alternative coping mechanisms like a walk, meditation, or calling a friend.
**Eating Out of Habit:** Always grab a snack at 3 PM? Maybe it's just a ritual rather than actual hunger. Try replacing it with a non-food habit, like stretching or deep breathing.

## 6. The Beauty of Distraction

Believe it or not, engaging in an activity can often lessen or even erase the sensation of hunger. Read a book, paint, dance, or dive into a hobby. Engage your mind, and you'll be amazed at how often hunger takes a backseat.

## 7. Hydrate, Hydrate, Hydrate

Often, our bodies confuse thirst with hunger. Before reaching for a snack, drink a glass of water. Herbal teas or infused waters can also be delightful allies in your fasting journey.

## 8. Celebrate Small Wins

Did you wait out a hunger pang and realize it faded after a while? Celebrate that! Acknowledging these moments reinforces positive behavior, making it easier over time.

## 9. Seeking Support

Discussing your feelings about hunger with supportive friends, family, or fasting communities can be incredibly therapeutic. Sharing experiences, seeking advice, or simply venting can make the journey less intimidating.

## 10. Be Gentle with Yourself

Last, but by no means least, remember to be kind to yourself. Overcoming the fear of hunger is a journey, not a destination. There'll be days when you'll navigate it with grace, and days when the chocolate cake wins. And that's perfectly okay.

## In Closing...

Hunger, in many ways, is like an old song, evoking a cascade of emotions and memories. By tuning into our bodies, understanding the roots of our fears, and employing strategies to address them, we can learn to dance to this song rather than resist it.

So, the next time your stomach gives that familiar grumble, smile. It's just singing you a song, reminding you of the incredible, adaptive, and resilient being you are.

# Chapter 15: Emotional and Psychological Aspects
## Part III: Mindful Eating

Let's take a moment to imagine. You're seated at a table, your favorite dish in front of you, a gentle aroma wafting towards you. Instead of diving right in, you pause. You inhale deeply, appreciating the scent. You marvel at the colors, textures, and the love that went into preparing this meal. Then, with gratitude, you take your first bite, savoring every nuance of flavor. This, dear reader, is the essence of mindful eating.

### 1. What is Mindful Eating?

Mindful eating is like meditation, but centered around our food. It's about being present during meals, relishing each bite, and tuning into our body's signals. It's not just about what we eat, but how we eat.

### 2. Why Mindful Eating Matters

In today's world, multitasking has become our second nature. How often have we eaten a meal while scrolling on our phones, watching TV, or even driving? The downside? We miss out on the joy of the eating experience, often overeat, and are left feeling unsatisfied.

When we eat mindfully:

- We appreciate our food more.
- We recognize our body's hunger and fullness cues.
- Digestion improves as we eat slower and chew thoroughly.

### 3. The Connection with Fasting

You might wonder, "We've been talking about fasting. How does eating fit in?" The beauty of fasting is the heightened sense of appreciation it brings to meals. When you finally break your fast, employing mindful eating can transform the experience from a simple meal to a profound moment of connection with your body and the food you consume.

## 4. Steps to Practice Mindful Eating

Let's embark on this delicious journey:

**Gratitude First:** Before you start, express gratitude. Think of the farmers, the chef, or even the universe that made this meal possible.

**Distraction-Free Zone:** Turn off the TV, put away the phone, and find a quiet place to eat. Let this be your 'me-time'.

**The Art of Observation:** Before you dive in, observe. What colors do you see? Can you identify the ingredients? Is your mouth watering yet?

**Savor Every Bite:** Place a small bite on your fork or spoon. When you place it in your mouth, resist the urge to swallow immediately. Taste it. Is it sweet? Salty? Spicy? Celebrate the complexity of flavors.

**Chew Thoroughly:** Did you know digestion begins in the mouth? Chewing not only helps break down food but also gives time for your body to signal when it's full.

**Tune into Your Senses:** What does the food feel like? What sounds do you hear as you chew? Engage all your senses in the act of eating.

**Pause Between Bites:** Put down your utensils between bites. This gives you time to truly savor what you've eaten and prepares you for the next delicious morsel.

**Check-in with Your Hunger:** Halfway through, stop and ask yourself, "Am I still hungry?" Your body knows best when it's had enough, and all it asks is for you to listen.

**Hydration is Key:** Often, our bodies can confuse thirst with hunger. Take sips of water during your meal to aid digestion and stay hydrated.

**Slow Down:** It's not a race! By slowing down, you'll likely find that you eat less but feel more satisfied.

### 5. Overcoming Challenges

Mindful eating might seem daunting at first. "I don't have time for this," or "It sounds too spiritual," might be thoughts that come to mind. Remember, like any habit, it gets easier over time. And it's not about perfection; it's about experience. Some meals might be rushed, and that's okay. But aim to have at least one mindful meal a day.

### 6. The Bigger Picture: Mindful Living

Eating mindfully can be the first step towards living mindfully. It can teach you patience, gratitude, and the value of the present moment. These are lessons you can take with you beyond the dining table, into every aspect of your life.

### Closing Thoughts...

In the realm of fasting and nutrition, we often get caught up in the 'whats'—what to eat, what to avoid. But the 'hows'—how we eat, how we approach food—can be equally transformative.

Mindful eating isn't just a practice; it's an invitation—a gentle call to return to the present, to find joy in the little things, and to nurture a relationship of love and respect with our bodies. So the next time you sit down for a meal, remember: It's not just food on that plate; it's an experience waiting to be cherished.

# CHAPTER 16: TROUBLESHOOTING AND ADJUSTING PROTOCOLS

## Part I: Personalizing Your Fast

Alright, so you've journeyed into the world of fasting, learned the nuances, seen the wide array of benefits, and you might have even started experimenting with a few protocols. But here's the beautiful thing about our bodies – they're as unique as our fingerprints. Which means? No one-size-fits-all approach.

In this part, we're diving deep into personalizing your fast. Let's co-create a protocol that resonates with YOU.

### 1. Understand Why You're Fasting

Before altering or choosing any fasting protocol, circle back to your 'why'. Are you seeking:

Weight management?
Enhanced cognitive functions?
Digestive system reset?
Spiritual or mental clarity?

Your goals play a massive role in shaping your fasting journey.

## 2. Recognize Your Baseline

Think of your current state as a starting point on a map.

**Physical Aspects:** Consider factors like your weight, metabolic rate, activity level, and any prevailing health conditions.
**Emotional and Mental Aspects:** How's your relationship with food? Are you currently undergoing significant stress or emotional turmoil?

Recognizing where you are will help you decide which direction to take.

## 3. Flexibility is Your Friend

Look, life happens! There are holidays, birthdays, and those days when you just crave a midnight snack. The beauty of fasting lies in its adaptability. Remember:

**Skipping a Fast Isn't Failing:** If you miss a fast or break it earlier than planned, it's not a setback. It's a learning experience.
**Listen to Your Body:** Feeling too drained during a fast? Maybe it's time to adjust the duration or the type of fast.

## 4. Feedback Loop: The Body's Messaging Service

Your body is continually communicating with you. These signals can help you tweak your fasting protocol:

**Energy Levels:** If you're always fatigued during your fast, consider shortening the duration or adjusting the time.
**Hunger vs. Cravings:** Feeling hungry during a fast is natural. But if you're experiencing intense, consistent cravings, it might indicate nutrient deficiencies or the need to change your eating window.

## 5. Factor in Physical Activity

You might be someone who loves to hit the gym, take long walks, or do yoga. Here's how to sync your fasting with fitness:

**High-Intensity Workouts:** If you're into heavy lifting or high-intensity interval training, it might be beneficial to eat a protein-rich meal post your workout. Consider adjusting your fasting window accordingly.

**Low-Intensity or Rest Days:** These are ideal for longer fasts as your energy expenditure is lower.

## 6. Women, Your Cycle Matters!

Ladies, our monthly cycles play a significant role in how we experience fasting:

**Follicular Phase (Day 1-14):** During the first half of your cycle, energy levels are generally higher, making it a suitable time for longer or more frequent fasts.

**Luteal Phase (Day 15-28):** As we near our periods, we might feel more fatigued or hungry. It's okay to be gentler and reduce fasting durations during this time.

## 7. Daily Life and Routines

Are you a night owl or an early bird? Do you work late shifts? Your daily routine can influence your fasting windows:

**Morning Persons:** If you feel most energetic in the AM, consider having an early dinner and skipping breakfast.

**Night Owls:** You might want to skip morning meals and have a more substantial dinner.

## 8. Experiment and Evolve

One of the most exciting parts of fasting? The freedom to experiment:

**Vary Durations:** Try a 16-hour fast for a week, then maybe a 24-hour fast. See what feels right.

**Hybrid Models:** Combine intermittent fasting with occasional extended fasts for a dynamic approach.

**Keep a Journal:** Document your feelings, energy levels, and any insights during various fasting experiments. It's a goldmine of personal data.

**9. Remember, It's Personal**

Dear reader, while guides (like this one), expert opinions, and research are great starting points, always remember that you're the ultimate expert on your body. Trust your intuition, embrace the journey, and relish the self-discovery.

**In Closing...**

Embarking on a personalized fasting journey is akin to crafting a masterpiece. It's a dance between science, intuition, and personal experience. So, as you chart out your unique path, know that every twist, turn, and pivot is a brushstroke on this beautiful canvas of self-awareness.

And hey, give yourself a pat on the back. You're not just following a trend; you're creating a tailor-made journey towards better health and self-understanding. Cheers to that!

# Chapter 16: Troubleshooting and Adjusting Protocols
## Part II: Recognizing Plateaus

Ah, plateaus. The proverbial peaks that seem to stand in the way of our journey, challenging our perseverance. Whether you've been fasting for a while or are just beginning, it's entirely possible you might hit one of these flat patches where it feels like nothing is moving forward. But fret not; plateaus are a natural part of any journey, especially one as transformative as fasting. Let's dive deep into understanding, recognizing, and ultimately breaking through these plateaus.

### 1. What Exactly is a Plateau?

In the world of health and fitness, a plateau typically refers to a period where you stop seeing progress despite your consistent efforts. This could mean no weight loss, no visible changes in physique, or not feeling the benefits you once did when you started fasting.

### 2. Why Do Plateaus Happen?

Understanding the 'why' can often be the key to unlocking the 'how' in solving a problem. So, let's get to the root of it:

**Adaptation:** Our bodies are wondrously adaptive. When you begin a new regimen like fasting, your body initially responds because it's a change from the norm. But with time, it adjusts and the rate of change slows down.

**Metabolic Rate Changes:** As you lose weight, your body requires fewer calories. This means the deficit between calories consumed and burned reduces, slowing down weight loss.

**Inconsistent Fasting Protocols:** Sometimes, the issue can be inconsistency. If you're not sticking to your fasting protocols or are often breaking them, it might lead to a plateau.

### 3. Signs You've Hit a Plateau

While weight is the most common metric, it's not the only indicator of a plateau. Here are some signs:

**Static Weight:** You've maintained a consistent weight despite sticking to your fasting regimen.

**Energy Levels:** You no longer feel that surge of energy or mental clarity you did when you started fasting.

**Hunger Pangs:** Previously manageable hunger pangs might become more pronounced, making it hard to stick to the fast.

**Emotional Indicators:** Feelings of frustration, demotivation, or a drop in mood can also be signs. Remember, our bodies and minds are deeply connected.

### 4. Breaking Through the Plateau

If you've identified that you're on a plateau, take a moment to commend yourself. Recognition is the first step to action. Now, let's explore some steps to move past it:

**Reassess Your Goals:** It's a great time to revisit and refine your goals. Maybe your initial goal was weight loss, but now it's more about maintaining muscle tone or improving digestion. Be clear on what you want.

**Change It Up:** The saying "Variety is the spice of life" holds here. Consider varying your fasting windows, trying a different fasting method, or even incorporating a few days of mindful eating without fasting.

**Calorie Cycling:** Instead of consuming the same number of calories every day, consider cycling them. Consume more calories on some days and fewer on others. This can jolt your system and kickstart progress.

**Re-evaluate Your Diet:** Are you consuming nutrient-dense foods during your eating windows? Sometimes the quality of calories matters more than the quantity.

**Stay Active:** If you aren't already, incorporate regular physical activity into your routine. If you are, perhaps it's time to intensify or vary your workouts.

**Mind Over Body:** Meditation, positive affirmations, or even joining a community can help combat the emotional effects of a plateau.

## 5. Things to Keep in Mind

**Be Patient:** Rome wasn't built in a day, and neither is the best version of you. Understand that plateaus, like any challenge, are temporary.

**Avoid Over-Compensation:** It might be tempting to drastically cut calories or over-exercise, but this can do more harm than good. Remember, balance is key.

**Seek Support:** Talk to others in the fasting community, consider seeking advice from a nutritionist, or even chat with friends and family. Sometimes an outside perspective can offer invaluable insights.

## Closing Thoughts…

If there's one thing I'd like you to take away, it's this: plateaus are not dead ends. They're simply pauses, moments for reflection, and potentially even redirection. Every person's fasting journey is unique, and challenges are bound to arise. But with patience, perseverance, and perhaps a pinch of creativity, you can navigate these plateaus and continue on your path to holistic wellness.

Always remember, fasting isn't just a physical endeavor. It's a dance between mind, body, and spirit. And sometimes, in any dance, we take a step back to leap forward even stronger.

## Chapter 16: Troubleshooting and Adjusting Protocols
## Part III: Addressing Specific Health Concerns

Alright, my fellow fasting enthusiast, we've danced through the technical bits, recognized plateaus, and now, it's time for an important tango: addressing specific health concerns. While fasting holds a bouquet of benefits, it's essential to be aware and cautious, especially if you have underlying health issues. So let's waltz through this together, step by step.

**1. Fasting and Diabetes**

First on our list, and perhaps one of the most talked-about concerns, is diabetes.

**Type 1 Diabetes:** For those with Type 1 diabetes, fasting can be tricky. It's vital to monitor blood sugar levels closely as fasting can lead to low blood sugar (hypoglycemia). Always consult with a healthcare professional before diving into a fasting routine.

**Type 2 Diabetes:** Intermittent fasting may offer benefits, such as improving insulin sensitivity. However, like our friends with Type 1, vigilance is key. Regularly check your blood sugar and ensure you're eating balanced meals during your eating window.

**2. Fasting and Heart Health**

The heart – the very drumbeat of our existence!

**High Blood Pressure:** Some studies suggest that fasting might help lower blood pressure. But, if you're on medication, the combo of fasting and meds might drop it too low. A doctor's guidance here is essential.

**Cholesterol:** While fasting might help improve cholesterol levels for some, others might experience a rise, especially in LDL (the not-so-great cholesterol). Regular check-ups will help you understand how fasting impacts you individually.

**3. Fasting and Thyroid Issues**

Ah, the thyroid, our metabolic maestro!

**Hypothyroidism:** Fasting can sometimes exacerbate hypothyroid symptoms, making you feel more fatigued. It's essential to monitor how you feel and consult with an endocrinologist.

**Hyperthyroidism:** On the flip side, with hyperthyroidism, your metabolism is already in overdrive. Fasting might add extra stress to your body. Again, monitoring and doctor consultation is the way to go.

### 4. Fasting and Digestive Disorders

The gut – our second brain, and a central player in our well-being.

**IBS and IBD:** Fasting can sometimes relieve symptoms of Irritable Bowel Syndrome and Inflammatory Bowel Disease by giving the gut a break. But, and this is a big but, for some, it might trigger symptoms. It's a bit of a tightrope walk, so having a gastroenterologist in your corner can be super helpful.

**Acid Reflux:** If you're prone to heartburn or GERD, fasting might exacerbate symptoms, especially if you end up consuming larger meals or spicy foods during your eating window. Keep a food diary to pinpoint triggers.

### 5. Fasting and Hormonal Imbalances

The delicate symphony of hormones! They play such a pivotal role in our mood, energy, and overall health.

**PCOS:** Women with Polycystic Ovary Syndrome might benefit from the insulin-regulating effects of fasting. But be cautious; fasting can also impact menstrual cycles. If you have PCOS and are considering fasting, it's a conversation worth having with your gynecologist.

**Adrenal Fatigue:** Stressing an already stressed system? Not the best idea. If you suffer from adrenal fatigue, prolonged fasting might not be your best buddy. Listen to your body, and remember: there's no one-size-fits-all.

**6. Fasting and Chronic Illnesses**

From autoimmune disorders to chronic fatigue syndrome, the effects of fasting can vary. The golden rule? You guessed it – monitor and consult with a specialist.

**Closing Thoughts...**

Remember this: fasting is a tool, not a magic wand. Its impact can be profoundly positive, but it also demands respect, especially when health concerns come into play. Embrace fasting as a journey of learning – about the world, about wellness, but most importantly, about yourself.

Your body is the most incredible instrument you'll ever own. Sometimes it's a gentle harp, sometimes a roaring guitar, but it's always playing the song of you. So, in every chord, every note, and every rest, listen intently. It will tell you what it needs, when to push forward, and when to pause.

And remember, whether you're dancing through plateaus or navigating the melodies of specific health concerns, you're never truly alone on this journey. We're all in this beautiful, intricate dance of life together.

# CHAPTER 17: COMBINING FASTING WITH OTHER DIETS

## Part I: Ketogenic Diet

Ah, the ketogenic diet - a term that has buzzed around the wellness world like a busy little bee. And you might be wondering, "Can I pair this fat-loving diet with fasting?" Well, my friend, you're in for a treat. Let's dive deep into the world of ketosis and see how it dances harmoniously with fasting. Grab your dance shoes, and let's twirl into the keto realm!

**What's the Keto Buzz All About?**

In its simplest form, the ketogenic (or keto) diet is a high-fat, moderate-protein, and low-carb diet. It shifts your body's fuel source from glucose (sugar) to ketones (compounds made when the body breaks down fats). So instead of relying on that pasta bowl for energy, your body turns to its fat stores, essentially making you a fat-burning machine.

**The Synergy of Keto and Fasting**

Keto and fasting are like two peas in a pod. They both aim to deplete the body's glucose reserves to tap into those glorious ketones for energy. When combined:

1. **Accelerated Ketosis:** Fasting can help you enter ketosis

quicker. Ever felt that energy surge after not eating for a while? That's your body hinting at ketosis.

**2. Enhanced Fat Burning:** When already in ketosis from a keto diet, fasting can rev up the fat-burning process. It's like adding a turbo booster!

**3. Autophagy Boost:** Both fasting and keto can stimulate autophagy, the body's way of cleaning out damaged cells and regenerating new ones. It's like spring cleaning but for your cells.

## How to Dance the Keto-Fasting Waltz

Merging keto with fasting can feel overwhelming. It's like learning new dance steps. So, here are some steps to waltz gracefully into the world of keto-fasting:

**1. Ease Into It:** If you're new to both, start with one. Get comfortable with keto first, understanding how your body reacts to reduced carbs. Once you're keto-adapted, weave in fasting.

**2. Stay Hydrated:** With decreased carbs, water retention drops, and you might get dehydrated. Drink up! And don't forget those electrolytes; they're crucial, especially sodium, magnesium, and potassium.

**3. Fat is Your Friend:** Don't shy away from healthy fats. Avocados, nuts, seeds, coconut oil, and fatty fish should be on your go-to list. They'll be your primary energy source.

**4. Mind Your Protein:** On keto, protein is moderate, not high. Too much protein can kick you out of ketosis. Aim for quality sources like grass-fed beef, free-range eggs, and wild-caught fish.

**5. Vegetable Game Strong:** Even though carbs are limited, green leafy veggies should grace your plate regularly. They're low in carbs but high in fiber and essential nutrients.

**6. Choose Your Fasting Window:** If you're intermittent fasting, decide on a window that suits you. The 16:8 (16 hours of fasting and an 8-hour eating window) is popular among keto-fasters.

**7. Listen to Your Body:** This can't be emphasized enough. Keto-flu (a group of symptoms that might appear when starting keto) is real, and so is fasting fatigue. If you feel off, consider tweaking your approach.

**Common Hurdles (And How to Leap Over Them)**

Merging keto with fasting isn't always a smooth waltz. You might stumble on a few hurdles:

**1. Energy Lows:** Initially, as your body shifts from glucose to ketones, you might feel drained. Power through! It's temporary. Soon, you'll be riding the keto energy wave.

**2. Cravings:** Oh, the sweet siren call of carbs! Especially in the beginning, your body might scream for a piece of bread. Stay strong. Over time, as you become fat-adapted, these cravings usually diminish.

**3. Social Situations:** Dining out? Friends think you're in a weird "fat cult"? It can be challenging. Opt for salads with protein and fats when out. And as for friends, maybe share some keto-friendly dessert. Food always wins them over!

**4. Digestive Woes:** A sudden dive into fats might upset your tummy. Gradually increase your fat intake. And don't neglect fiber from veggies to keep things... well, moving.

**Wrapping Up Our Dance**

Combining the ketogenic diet with fasting is like performing a dance that celebrates the body's ability to adapt and thrive. When done with care, understanding, and a dash of patience, it can be a transformative experience.

Remember, though, the dance floor of health and wellness is

vast. This keto-fasting waltz is but one dance among many. So while it's okay to groove to the keto beat, always ensure it aligns with your body's rhythm. Dance on, my friend, dance on!

# Chapter 17: Combining Fasting with Other Diets
## Part II: Mediterranean Diet

Oh, the Mediterranean! Just hearing the word, I bet you can almost feel the warm sun kissing your skin, the gentle breeze with a hint of salt from the azure sea, and the tantalizing aroma of fresh olives and grilled fish wafting through the air. Isn't it enchanting? Now, imagine encapsulating that essence into a diet. That, dear reader, is the Mediterranean diet for you.

## Why the Mediterranean Diet is So Loved

First things first. Let's unwrap the gift that is the Mediterranean diet.

The Mediterranean diet isn't just a "diet". It's more a lifestyle, inspired by the traditional eating habits of countries like Spain, Italy, and Greece. The focus? Fresh, seasonal, and local produce, heart-healthy fats, and an active lifestyle.

It's brimming with veggies, fruits, legumes, nuts, and whole grains. Seafood has a starring role, while poultry, eggs, and dairy make guest appearances. Red meat? It's in there too, but more like a rare cameo. And let's not forget that little glass of red wine!

## The Beautiful Fusion of the Mediterranean Diet and Fasting

Now, how does this sunny diet fit into our fasting puzzle? Beautifully, as it turns out. The Mediterranean diet is rich in nutrients yet moderate in calories, making it a perfect companion for fasting. Here's why:

**1. Nutrient Density:** With fasting, your eating window might shrink, but your body's need for nutrients doesn't. The Mediterranean diet, abundant in vitamins, minerals, and antioxidants, ensures you're not shortchanged.

**2. Heart-Healthy Fats:** Olive oil, nuts, and fish offer omega-3 fatty acids and monounsaturated fats. These can help reduce inflammation – a lovely complement to fasting's anti-inflammatory benefits.

**3. Gentle on Blood Sugar:** This diet is naturally low in processed foods and sugars, ensuring a stable blood sugar level, which syncs well with fasting's goal of insulin regulation.

**4. Flexibility:** It's easy to adjust. On non-fasting days, enjoy a more abundant spread. On fasting days, reduce portions but maintain the nutrient diversity.

**Dancing the Mediterranean-Fasting Tango**

Let's choreograph our dance steps to blend the Mediterranean diet with fasting:

**1. Start Slowly:** If you're new to the Mediterranean diet, ease in. Swap butter for olive oil, introduce more fish into your diet, and incorporate more fruits and veggies.

**2. Plan Your Plates:** During your eating windows, aim for a plate that's half veggies, a quarter protein (like fish or legumes), and a quarter whole grains. Drizzle with some olive oil and perhaps a sprinkle of feta.

**3. Hydration is Key:** While the Mediterranean diet is rich in water-filled veggies and fruits, remember to sip on water, herbal teas, and the occasional glass of red wine (in moderation, of course!).

**4. Diverse Protein Sources:** Benefit from the array of protein sources – legumes, fish, poultry. This ensures a well-rounded amino acid profile.

**5. Fast-Friendly Meals:** On fasting days, opt for lighter dishes like Greek salads, lentil soups, or grilled sardines.

**6. Mindful Eating:** Just as the Mediterranean lifestyle emphasizes enjoying meals with family and friends, practice being present. Savor each bite.

**7. Adapt as Needed:** Depending on your fasting schedule, tweak meal compositions. Longer fast? Prioritize protein and fats for satiety. Shorter fast? Maybe a touch more carbs for energy.

## Little Waves to Watch Out For

As you sail this Mediterranean-fasting journey, be aware of potential waves:

**1. Caloric Intake:** Olive oil, nuts, and avocados are nutrient-dense but also high in calories. Enjoy them, but be mindful of portions, especially if weight loss is a goal.

**2. Overcompensation:** After a fast, there might be a temptation to overindulge. Remember, it's about balance. Savor your meals, but don't binge.

**3. Alcohol Consumption:** While a glass of red wine is often hailed in this diet, it might not be for everyone, especially during fasting. Listen to your body.

**4. Social Settings:** Dining out? Opt for grilled fish, salads, or vegetable-centric dishes. Pass on the deep-fried or heavily processed options.

## Concluding Our Mediterranean Sojourn

Blending the Mediterranean diet with fasting is like enjoying a sun-soaked holiday for your cells. It's rejuvenating, refreshing, and deeply nourishing. And while every dance has its unique steps and rhythm, what truly matters is enjoying the journey.

Remember, the Mediterranean diet is not just about the food on your plate; it's about the joy in your heart, the laughter shared with loved ones, and the health you gain!

## Chapter 17: Combining Fasting with Other Diets
## Part III: Plant-based and Vegan Diets

It's fascinating how food journeys often reflect personal evolutions. From making choices based on taste, we've now shifted to making decisions based on health, ethics, and planetary impact. A significant chapter in many of these journeys is the exploration of plant-based and vegan diets.

I see you nodding. Whether you're just intrigued by it or have adopted it wholeheartedly, let's explore how fasting beautifully dovetails with these green, compassionate choices.

### Understanding Plant-based and Vegan Lifestyles

Before we dive in, let's get our definitions straight:

**Plant-based Diet:** Primarily focuses on consuming whole, minimally processed plants. It's not just about avoiding animal products but about emphasizing whole vegetables, fruits, nuts, seeds, oils, whole grains, legumes, and beans.

**Vegan Diet:** Goes a step beyond by eliminating all animal products, not just in diet but also in other areas like clothing and cosmetics, stemming from ethical, environmental, and health reasons.

### Merging Greens with Fasting: A Perfect Harmony

Plant-based and vegan diets, brimming with fiber and nutrients, align gracefully with fasting. Here's the harmonious duet they play:

**1. Natural Detoxification:** Both fasting and plant-based diets support the body's natural detoxification. When combined, this effect is amplified. Think of it as a double boost for your body's cleansing mechanism.

**2. Weight Management:** The fiber-richness of a plant-based diet ensures you feel full and satiated, complementing fasting's weight management benefits.

3. **Energy Efficiency:** Plants provide slow-releasing carbohydrates, ensuring steady energy, which is beneficial, especially when fasting.

4. **Reduced Inflammation:** Both fasting and plant-rich diets can reduce inflammation in the body. Together, they're like a soothing balm for your cells.

**Tips for Navigating the Plant-Based Fasting Pathway**

Embarking on this green-fast journey? Here are some signposts to guide you:

1. **Protein Puzzle:** One common concern is getting adequate protein. Fret not! Lentils, chickpeas, tofu, tempeh, seitan, quinoa, chia seeds, hemp seeds, and almonds are all excellent protein sources. Mix and match to ensure a complete amino acid profile.

2. **Mind Your Micronutrients:** While plants are nutrient powerhouses, certain nutrients like B12, Vitamin D, Omega-3 (usually from fish), and iron might need more attention. Plan wisely or consider supplements.

3. **Fasting-friendly Meals:** Opt for nutrient-dense, calorie-light meals. Think spinach and tofu salads, lentil soups, or a vegetable stir-fry with quinoa.

4. **Stay Hydrated:** Plant-based diets naturally contain a lot of water. Still, when fasting, up your hydration game with water, herbal teas, and natural, fresh juices (in moderation).

5. **Gradual Transition:** If you're new to plant-based eating, take it slow. Gradually increase plant-based days in your week, allowing your body to adjust.

6. **Ethical Synergy:** If you're drawn to veganism for ethical reasons, you'll find that fasting aligns with this ethos. It's about

mindfulness and conscious choices, not just about what you eat, but when and why.

**Tread with Awareness**

While the plant-based fasting path is paved with numerous benefits, there are areas to be conscious of:

**1. Nutrient Deficiency:** Regularly monitor levels of critical nutrients, especially if you're excluding all animal products. Consider periodic check-ups to ensure everything's on track.

**2. Listen to Your Body:** Especially during prolonged fasts, if you feel dizzy, fatigued, or unusually irritable, it might be a sign that you're missing out on some essential nutrients. Be responsive.

**3. Social Scenarios:** Eating out or at social gatherings might need a tad more planning. Call ahead at restaurants or consider having a small meal before heading out, so you're not starving when faced with limited choices.

**Concluding the Green Chapter**

Uniting the world of plant-based or vegan diets with fasting is akin to merging two beautiful philosophies. Both are about listening to your body, respecting all living beings, and making mindful choices.

So, as you venture into this verdant territory, remember it's more than just about the food on your plate. It's a holistic dance of health, ethics, and environmental responsibility. Embrace it with an open heart, let curiosity be your guide, and remember that every meal is an opportunity to make a choice that honors both your body and the planet.

# CHAPTER 18: REAL-LIFE TESTIMONIES

## Part I: Weight Loss Stories

It's easy to get caught up in scientific jargon, nutritional charts, and statistical results. But you know what speaks volumes? Real-life stories. They're the heartbeat that pumps life into data and statistics. Here, in this chapter, we'll dive deep into personal journeys of transformation, starting with the powerful narratives centered on weight loss.

I've always believed that every weight loss journey, just like every individual, is unique. So, I invite you to walk in the shoes of three brave souls who have found solace and success through fasting.

**Sarah's Journey: From Despair to Dancing**

"I never believed I'd say this, but fasting made me fall in love with myself again."

Sarah, a 34-year-old mother of two, found herself trapped in a cycle of emotional eating after her second child. With each passing day, she felt further from her former lively self and closer to the label of 'just a mom.'

She stumbled upon intermittent fasting accidentally during a late-night search for weight loss remedies. With a skeptical heart but desperate desire, she decided to give the 16:8 method a try.

The first week was tough. "I won't sugarcoat it," she says, "I was irritable and dreamt of bagels every night." But by week three, she felt a shift. Not just in her weight, but her energy levels. "It's like someone had turned on the light," she described.

In a year, Sarah lost 40 pounds. But more than the weight, she regained her confidence. "I dance now," she laughed, "in my living room, with my kids. I'm not 'just a mom' anymore; I'm a dancing queen."

**Raj's Redemption: Breaking Stereotypes**

"Being overweight in my community was a sign of prosperity. Little did they know how much I was suffering inside."

Raj grew up in an environment where a hefty physique was celebrated, a sign of wealth and abundance. But by his late 20s, Raj realized that his weight, which had once been a source of pride, was now a prison.

The societal pressures, combined with a high-stress job, led Raj to comfort eating. Fasting seemed alien, almost punitive to him. But a chance encounter with a nutritionist at a friend's party changed everything.

She introduced him to alternate-day fasting. "The idea seemed daunting," Raj confessed, "but there was something in her conviction that made me want to try."

The journey was challenging. There were moments of doubt, days of relapse. But Raj persisted. He combined fasting with daily walks, focusing on one step at a time. Sixteen months later, Raj was 60 pounds lighter.

But for him, the real victory was breaking free from the societal mold. "I've redefined prosperity for myself," he said, eyes shining, "It's not about looking affluent; it's about feeling alive."

## Lila's Leap: A Late Bloomer's Triumph

"They say it's harder to lose weight when you're older. I say, watch me."

At 58, Lila had almost accepted her expanding waistline as a byproduct of aging. Every family gathering was a reminder that she was the 'chubby aunt,' a tag she wore with reluctant resignation.

Her introduction to fasting was through a book gifted by her niece. "I was intrigued but skeptical," she recalls. She began with a gentler approach: the 12:12 method, fasting for 12 hours, and eating during the next 12.

Lila faced her fair share of naysayers. "Many said I was too old, that I was setting myself up for disappointment," she shared. But she quietly pressed on.

Lila's consistency bore fruit. She lost 30 pounds over two years. More than rapid weight loss, it was the newfound vitality that she cherished. "I garden now, something I hadn't done in a decade. I feel rooted, in more ways than one."

## Conclusion

Every weight loss story, including Sarah's, Raj's, and Lila's, is a testament to human resilience, hope, and the transformative power of fasting. But remember, dear reader, while weight loss can be a beautiful byproduct, the real win is in the renewed relationship with oneself. The number on the scale will never be as crucial as the glow in one's eyes or the spring in one's step. As you embark or continue on your journey, may you find your unique story of transformation.

# Chapter 18: Real-Life Testimonies
## Part II: Health Recovery Tales

While shedding extra pounds can be exhilarating, many people turn to fasting in hopes of revitalizing their health. Fasting, for many, isn't just a route to a slimmer body but a path to a healthier life, inside and out. In this segment, we'll delve into captivating accounts of individuals who've embraced fasting and, in the process, witnessed transformative health improvements.

### Alejandro's Awakening: From Fatigued to Fiery

"You know something's wrong when getting out of bed feels like climbing Everest," Alejandro quipped.

In his early 40s, Alejandro was diagnosed with Type 2 Diabetes. The constant fatigue, persistent thirst, and unending worry became his daily companions. Every meal became a math problem, and every sugar spike, a defeat.

He'd heard about the potential benefits of fasting for blood sugar regulation. "What did I have to lose?" he thought. Starting with short, 14-hour daily fasts, he gradually worked his way up to 20 hours.

The first noticeable change? "Energy! I felt like I was 20 again!" Alejandro exclaimed. With time, his blood sugar levels became more stable, and his medication was adjusted. "Fasting didn't just help my diabetes, it rekindled my zest for life."

### Celine's Comeback: Calming the Storm Within

"My body felt like it was at war with itself," Celine softly shared, remembering her battle with autoimmune conditions.

Struggling with Hashimoto's and rheumatoid arthritis, Celine's day was dictated by her flare-ups. The pain, inflammation, and brain fog made even simple tasks daunting. Numerous medications provided temporary relief, but Celine yearned for a lasting solution.

Her research led her to prolonged fasting. Initially apprehensive, she began with supervised, three-day fasts, gradually increasing their duration. "It wasn't easy, but it felt intuitive," she reflected.

Months into her fasting journey, Celine observed reduced inflammation and lesser flare-ups. "It was as if my body was resetting, recalibrating," she mused. Today, Celine champions fasting not just for its physical benefits, but for the mental clarity and emotional balance it brought her.

**Omari's Odyssey: Breaking Free from Digestive Woes**

"Imagine planning your life around the nearest restroom," Omari chuckled, "That was me!"

Battling Irritable Bowel Syndrome (IBS) since his teens, Omari's life was a tapestry of dietary restrictions, sudden flare-ups, and social awkwardness. Dates, travel, even casual outings were dictated by his unpredictable gut.

Upon a friend's recommendation, he ventured into intermittent fasting, specifically the 16:8 method. The results? "Life-changing," in Omari's words. He noticed fewer IBS episodes, reduced bloating, and an overall improved gut health.

"What surprised me the most was the newfound freedom," Omari confessed. "Freedom from worry, freedom to explore, to live spontaneously." Today, Omari is an avid traveler, with his gut woes no longer steering the wheel.

**Hana's Healing: The Battle against Hormonal Havoc**

"It felt like being on a never-ending roller coaster," Hana reflected on her struggle with Polycystic Ovary Syndrome (PCOS).

Erratic menstrual cycles, weight gain, acne, and mood swings - Hana's life was in constant upheaval. Tired of temporary fixes, she stumbled upon the potential benefits of fasting for hormonal balance.

She opted for a cyclic approach, syncing her fasting patterns with her menstrual cycle. "It felt harmonious, like I was dancing in tandem with my body," she described.

Over time, Hana noticed improved menstrual regularity, reduced symptoms, and, most importantly, a sense of empowerment. "Fasting didn't just regulate my hormones; it strengthened my bond with my body."

**Conclusion**

These accounts underscore the profound impact fasting can have beyond weight loss. From diabetes and autoimmune conditions to digestive and hormonal disorders, the healing potential of fasting touches various facets of health. But always remember, each journey is personal. What works for Alejandro, Celine, Omari, or Hana may not work for you. Yet, their stories remind us of the transformative power of resilience and the beauty of finding a path that resonates with our unique selves. As you navigate your own health odyssey, may you find your rhythm, your healing, and your testimony.

# Chapter 18: Real-Life Testimonies
## Part III: Psychological and Emotional Transformations

When we think of fasting, the immediate connections are often physical: weight loss, metabolic shifts, and detoxification. But the realm of fasting extends beyond the tangible and ventures into the profound territories of our minds and hearts. This section sheds light on the psychological and emotional rebirths experienced by those who have embraced fasting. Their tales are as diverse as they are, yet they all echo a common theme: transformation.

### Ella's Euphoria: From Clouds to Clarity

"I felt like I was constantly wading through mental fog," Ella started, "Every thought was an effort, every decision, a battle."

Struggling with anxiety and occasional bouts of depression, Ella's mental world was a maze of apprehensions and uncertainties. Then, her friend suggested intermittent fasting as a potential remedy. Although skeptical, Ella gave it a shot, adopting a 16:8 approach.

Weeks into her new routine, Ella began to experience moments of unprecedented mental clarity. "It was as if the fog had lifted, revealing a landscape I never knew existed," she described, her eyes sparkling. Over time, this clarity extended to her emotional world, helping her better understand and manage her feelings.

Today, Ella credits fasting for her mental rejuvenation. While it didn't erase her challenges, it certainly equipped her with a sharper mind and a resilient heart to navigate them.

### Jared's Journey: Rediscovering Self-Worth

Jared's story begins with a heartbreak. A failed relationship that left him questioning his self-worth and plunging into the depths of low self-esteem. The negative self-talk became incessant, and Jared felt trapped in his own mind.

A documentary on fasting serendipitously caught his attention, and it spoke of the spiritual and emotional aspects of this age-old practice. Motivated to give it a try, Jared embarked on periodic 24-hour fasts.

The first few attempts were a struggle, not just physically but emotionally. But with each completed fast, Jared felt a sense of accomplishment that slowly chipped away at his self-doubt. The hunger pangs transitioned into moments of introspection, where he confronted and began healing his emotional wounds.

Months later, Jared emerged with renewed self-worth and confidence. "Fasting wasn't just about abstaining from food; it was about feasting on self-love," he reflected.

**Priya's Passage: Embracing the Present**

"I was either agonizing over the past or dreading the future. The present? It seemed non-existent," Priya candidly shared about her challenges with mindfulness.

Distracted and often overwhelmed, Priya's life was a whirlwind of tasks and worries. Her mental peace was always just out of reach until she discovered the benefits of fasting combined with meditation.

She began with short fasts, using the heightened alertness to engage in deep meditation. The hunger, instead of being a distraction, became an anchor to the present. "Every hunger pang was a gentle reminder to come back to the moment," Priya mused.

This practice transformed Priya's relationship with time. She became more present, appreciating the beauty in the now. Her anxieties receded, replaced by a serene acceptance of what is.

**Leon's Liberation: From Control to Surrender**

Leon was a self-proclaimed control freak. Every aspect of his life was meticulously planned, leaving no room for spontaneity. This need for control stemmed from deeper fears of uncertainty and change.

Hearing about the discipline required in fasting, Leon saw it as another challenge to conquer. But his fasting journey turned out to be more than he'd anticipated. The inability to control his body's reactions and the unpredictability of his energy levels initially frustrated him. Yet, over time, something shifted.

He began to see the beauty in surrender, in letting go of the incessant need to control. Fasting taught Leon the value of trust —trust in his body and the natural processes of life.

"It's funny," Leon chuckled, "I began fasting to exert control, but I continue it to embrace the freedom of letting go."

## Conclusion

The psychological and emotional landscapes are intricate, with deep-rooted patterns and beliefs. Yet, as these stories show, the act of fasting offers a unique avenue to touch and transform these depths. Whether it's clarity, self-worth, presence, or surrender, the fasting journey is as much about nourishing the soul as it is about the body. And in these tales, we find not just testimonies, but invitations—to embark on our own journey of inner transformation.

# CHAPTER 19: TIPS FOR LONG-TERM SUCCESS

## Part I: Staying Motivated

The journey of fasting is akin to running a marathon rather than a sprint. Like any endurance activity, staying motivated is essential. The benefits of fasting can be life-changing, but reaching that pinnacle of success requires dedication, commitment, and most importantly, motivation.

So, how do you keep the fire of motivation burning, even when the going gets tough? Let's dive into the heart of staying motivated during your fasting journey.

**1. Revisit Your 'Why'**

Do you remember the day you decided to start fasting? There was a reason, a 'why'. Perhaps it was to shed some weight, gain mental clarity, or embark on a journey of self-discovery. This 'why' is your anchor.

Whenever you feel your motivation waning, close your eyes and revisit that moment. Visualize your goals and the reasons behind them. Understanding and reminding yourself of the bigger picture can reignite the passion and drive that got you started.

## 2. Celebrate Small Wins

While it's important to keep your eyes on the ultimate goal, don't forget to celebrate the milestones along the way. Did you complete a 16-hour fast for the first time? That's a win! Did you resist the temptation of breaking your fast early? Another win!

Every small victory is a step closer to your ultimate goal. By acknowledging and celebrating these achievements, you generate positive reinforcement, making the journey enjoyable.

## 3. Connect with a Community

The path of fasting can sometimes feel lonely, especially if those around you don't share or understand your journey. This is where a community comes into play. Connect with fellow fasters – whether it's online forums, social media groups, or local meet-ups. Sharing experiences, challenges, and successes with like-minded individuals can provide the encouragement you need to stay on track.

## 4. Educate Yourself

Knowledge is power. The more you understand about fasting, its benefits, and the science behind it, the more motivated you'll be to continue. Read books, attend seminars, or listen to podcasts on fasting. As you expand your knowledge, your commitment to the practice deepens.

## 5. Listen to Your Body

Your body is constantly communicating with you. Listen to it. If you feel genuinely fatigued or unwell, it might be an indication to adjust your fasting schedule or method. By being in tune with your body's needs and adjusting accordingly, you maintain a positive relationship with fasting, which is crucial for long-term motivation.

## 6. Keep a Journal

Documenting your journey can be incredibly motivating. Start a fasting journal where you note down your daily experiences, feelings, and realizations. Over time, this journal will become a testament to your growth, challenges overcome, and the myriad benefits you've experienced. On days when motivation seems hard to find, flipping through your journal can offer the encouragement you need.

### 7. Set Realistic Expectations

While fasting offers numerous benefits, it's essential to set realistic expectations. Understand that results may vary. Some might experience rapid weight loss, while for others, the benefits could be more subtle and internal. By keeping your expectations grounded, you prevent potential disappointments which could derail your motivation.

### 8. Integrate Mindfulness Practices

Fasting isn't just about refraining from food; it's a holistic experience. Integrating mindfulness practices like meditation can enhance the fasting experience. Not only does it offer mental clarity, but it also strengthens your resolve and motivation to continue.

### 9. Seek Inspiration

Whether it's a motivational quote, a success story, or a documentary on the benefits of fasting, seeking external sources of inspiration can give you the motivational boost you need. Find what resonates with you and turn to it whenever you feel your enthusiasm dip.

### 10. Remember, It's Okay to Start Again

Every journey has its bumps. There might be days or even weeks when you stray from your fasting routine. And that's okay. What's essential is not the stumble but the willingness to stand up and start again. Every new day offers a fresh opportunity to recommit to your goals.

Staying motivated throughout your fasting journey is a blend of internal resolve and external support. By regularly revisiting your reasons, celebrating your progress, connecting with others, and continuously feeding your mind and soul with knowledge and inspiration, you lay the groundwork for long-term success. Remember, fasting is a journey of self-discovery, growth, and transformation. And every step, no matter how challenging, is worth the unparalleled rewards waiting at the finish line.

## Chapter 19: Tips for Long-term Success
## Part II: Tracking Progress

There's an old saying that goes, "What gets measured gets managed." This adage is particularly true when embarking on your fasting journey. Tracking progress isn't merely a record of your achievements; it serves as a beacon of encouragement, a validation of your efforts, and a roadmap for future directions.

But what's the most effective way to track progress? And why is it so essential? Join me as we explore the profound significance of keeping tabs on your journey and the best methods to do so.

### 1. The Power of Visual Documentation

Ever heard stories of individuals who didn't realize the weight they'd lost until they compared their before-and-after photos? There's something incredibly motivating about visual proof.

**Photos:** Take monthly photos of yourself from multiple angles in consistent lighting. Over time, these photos will piece together a visual narrative of your transformative journey. On days when the scale isn't budging or you're feeling a little disheartened, these photos can serve as a stark reminder of how far you've come.

### 2. Maintain a Fasting Diary

A fasting diary goes beyond recording the number of hours you've fasted. It delves into the heart of your experiences.

**Daily Entries:** Make it a habit to jot down not just the length of your fast, but also your energy levels, mood, and any specific challenges you encountered. Did you feel unusually hungry? Were you more energetic? These notes can help you discern patterns and adapt accordingly.

### 3. Use Technology to Your Advantage

We're living in a digital age, and there's an app for almost everything—including fasting.

**Fasting Apps:** Numerous apps today can help you set fasting goals, send reminders, and track your fasting periods. They often come with additional features, like community forums or educational resources. Such apps can serve as both an accountability partner and a source of inspiration.

## 4. Monitor Physiological Changes

Fasting can bring about a plethora of physiological changes, many of which can be tracked to gauge progress.

**Blood Work:** Consider getting periodic blood tests. Monitoring levels of cholesterol, blood sugar, and other vital markers can provide insights into the internal benefits of your fasting regimen.

**Weight and Measurements:** While weight is a common metric, it doesn't always provide the full picture, especially if you're also building muscle. Taking monthly body measurements can offer a more comprehensive view of your physical transformation.

## 5. Reflect on Emotional and Mental Shifts

The benefits of fasting aren't merely physical. Many individuals report significant emotional and mental shifts.

**Mood Tracking:** Consider keeping a mood chart. Over time, you might find that fasting improves your mental clarity, mood stability, or overall emotional well-being.

**Journaling:** Beyond a fasting diary, maintaining a personal journal can capture the deeper emotional and psychological shifts you undergo. It's not just about the body—it's about the holistic transformation of mind, body, and spirit.

## 6. Engage with a Support System

Sharing your journey with someone else can be immensely rewarding. This doesn't just mean updating them on your successes, but also discussing your challenges.

**Accountability Partner:** Having someone who's aware of your goals and checks in with you can make a world of difference. This person can celebrate with you during your highs and offer support during the lows.

**Join a Group:** Whether online or offline, joining a fasting community can be beneficial. Sharing experiences and milestones can keep you motivated and provide valuable insights.

### 7. Reassess and Set New Goals

As you progress on your fasting journey, it's vital to pause occasionally and reassess.

**Goal Setting:** Maybe you began with a 16-hour intermittent fasting goal and now feel ready to try a 24-hour fast. Continually setting and working towards new goals ensures you keep growing and prevents stagnation.

### 8. The Non-Physical Milestones

Not every achievement can be measured in pounds lost or inches trimmed. Sometimes, the most significant milestones are non-physical.

**Increased Energy:** Perhaps you now find yourself more energetic and less reliant on that mid-afternoon caffeine jolt.

**Improved Sleep:** Many fasters report deeper, more restful sleep. If you're waking up feeling more refreshed, that's a significant milestone in itself.

Remember, tracking your progress isn't just about validation; it's about reflection, adaptation, and inspiration. While the numbers and data provide one perspective, it's the amalgamation of physical, emotional, and psychological growth that paints the full picture. Your journey with fasting is unique, and every step—no matter how big or small—deserves to be acknowledged, celebrated, and used as a stepping stone for future growth. By keeping a close eye on your evolution, you're not only crafting a story of transformation but also setting the foundation for sustained, long-term success.

## Chapter 19: Tips for Long-term Success
## Part III: Reintroducing Foods After Fasting

If you've reached this point, kudos to you. Whether you've just completed a short intermittent fast or an extended multi-day journey, one thing's for sure: the way you reintroduce food into your system matters. It's like the curtain call after an elaborate stage performance; you want it to be just as graceful as the act itself.

### 1. The Art of Breaking a Fast

Coming out of a fast isn't as simple as diving into a sumptuous buffet (as tempting as that might sound). It's an art, and it's critical for your digestive system.

**Gentle Start:** After a fasting period, your digestive system has been on a bit of a vacation. Jumping straight into heavy, complex meals might be overwhelming. Start with something light like a broth, a smoothie, or a small piece of fruit.

### 2. Hydrate, Hydrate, Hydrate

Water is, as always, your best friend. But after fasting, hydration plays a more pivotal role than merely quenching thirst.

**Electrolyte Balance:** Extended fasting can affect your electrolyte balance. Rehydrating with an electrolyte solution or natural coconut water can help replenish lost minerals.
**Prepping the Gut:** Water can help gently prepare your stomach and intestines for the solid foods you're about to reintroduce.

### 3. Be Mindful of Portion Sizes

I get it. You might feel like you could eat a horse. But remember, your stomach has likely shrunk a bit during the fasting period.

**Small Meals:** Initially, consider having smaller, more frequent meals. This approach is gentler on the stomach and ensures you don't overburden your digestive system.

**Listen to Your Body:** As always, tune into your body's cues. It will let you know when it's satisfied.

### 4. The Role of Fiber

Fiber is fantastic for digestion. But after fasting, it's beneficial to reintroduce it slowly.

**Slow and Steady:** Start with softer, cooked veggies before gradually transitioning to raw ones.
**Beans and Legumes:** If these are part of your regular diet, reintroduce them gradually to avoid digestive discomfort.

### 5. Proteins and Fats: The Reintroduction

Proteins and fats are essential, but post-fasting, there's a method to the reintroduction madness.

**Lean Proteins:** Begin with easier-to-digest proteins like fish or tofu. Gradually, you can incorporate chicken, turkey, and red meats.
**Healthy Fats:** Avocados, olives, and nuts are great sources. But remember, moderation is key in the beginning.

### 6. Carbohydrates: Yes, But Choose Wisely

Carbs often get a bad rap, but they're essential for energy.

**Complex Carbs:** Quinoa, sweet potatoes, and brown rice are excellent choices. They release energy slowly, preventing sudden blood sugar spikes.
**Limit Sugars:** After a fast, it's especially crucial to limit simple sugars, as they can cause rapid blood sugar fluctuations.

### 7. Monitor Your Response

Everyone's body is unique. While one person might feel great reintroducing a particular food, it might not sit well with another.

**Food Journal:** Consider maintaining a food journal. It can help you note down any reactions or discomforts associated with specific foods.

Adjust Accordingly: If a particular food doesn't resonate with you, it's okay to eliminate it and try reintroducing it at a later time.

## 8. Mindful Eating: A Continuation

Remember our previous discussion on mindful eating? It's time to put that into practice, especially now.

**Chew Slowly:** Digestion starts in the mouth. Taking time to chew not only aids digestion but also enhances the appreciation of flavors.

**Gratitude:** Before you eat, take a moment to express gratitude. For the food, for your body's resilience, for this journey.

## 9. Expect Some Physical Reactions

It's not uncommon to experience some bloating, gas, or changes in bowel habits as you reintroduce foods.

**Stay Calm:** These reactions are typically temporary. However, if they persist, consider consulting with a healthcare professional.

**Probiotics:** Incorporating probiotic-rich foods like yogurt or fermented vegetables can aid in restoring gut balance.

## 10. The Emotional Aspect of Eating Again

You might find that breaking a fast brings up unexpected emotions. Relief, joy, anxiety – it's all part of the journey.

**Be Kind to Yourself:** This process is as much emotional as it is physical. Celebrate the milestones, be gentle with the setbacks, and remember, every meal is an opportunity to nourish not just the body, but also the soul.

Wrapping it up, reintroducing foods post-fasting is a beautiful blend of science, art, and self-awareness. It's an opportunity to reconnect with food, to appreciate its myriad flavors, textures, and aromas, and to recognize its role in our overall well-being.

# CHAPTER 20: CONCLUDING THOUGHTS

## Part I: The Lifelong Journey

I can't help but start this concluding section with a simple yet profound acknowledgment: **you did it**. Regardless of where you are on this journey, whether at the start, in the midst, or reflecting after years of intermittent fasting, simply engaging with this process is an accomplishment in itself. It's worth celebrating.

When we began this book, the overarching goal was not just to introduce you to fasting, but to walk beside you, hand in hand, as you navigated its winding paths. Just as every winding path has its unique twists and turns, each person's fasting journey is inherently individual. This journey is as much about self-discovery as it is about health and wellness.

**1. The Ever-evolving Relationship with Food**

Your relationship with food, much like any relationship, is dynamic. It evolves, shifts, grows, and sometimes even stumbles. But it's precisely these fluctuations that make it alive, tangible, and profoundly personal.

With the tools and insights you've gathered from these pages, you're now equipped to navigate this relationship with greater mindfulness, understanding, and love. And remember, it's perfectly okay for this relationship to change over time. Life is fluid, and your approach to nourishment should be as well.

## 2. Beyond Physical Health

When we set out on this journey, the benefits of fasting, especially those tied to physical health, might have been the primary attraction. Weight loss, improved metabolic health, and heightened energy levels are undeniably compelling.

However, as you've hopefully discovered, fasting extends its embrace well beyond the physical realm. The psychological, emotional, and spiritual transformations that come with it are just as, if not more, transformative. This holistic wellness is the true essence of the fasting journey.

## 3. Embracing Imperfections

Let's be real for a moment. There might have been, or will be, days when you slip, days when the fast doesn't go as planned, or days when cravings seem insurmountable. And that's okay. Such moments don't define failure; they define humanity.

Each stumble is an opportunity—a chance to learn, adapt, and grow. It's essential to approach these moments not with self-judgment but with kindness and understanding. After all, this journey is about nurturing yourself.

## 4. Community and Support

No journey, no matter how personal, is solely a solitary endeavor. Along the way, you've likely encountered fellow travelers, each with their stories, insights, and experiences. This community, whether it's an online forum, a local group, or just a friend who shares your interest, is invaluable.

Lean on them. Share your victories, your challenges, and your insights. Remember, while the fasting journey is personal, the collective wisdom and encouragement of a supportive community can be an immense source of strength.

**5. The Dance of Flexibility**

The world of fasting, with its myriad protocols, guidelines, and recommendations, offers a framework. But the true magic lies in personalizing this framework to suit your unique rhythm.

Listen to your body, adjust when necessary, and allow yourself the flexibility to dance within the guidelines. Your body is wise, and it will guide you. Trust it.

**6. Lifelong Learning**

The realm of health and wellness, including fasting, is ever-evolving. New research emerges, fresh insights come to light, and our understanding deepens over time. Stay curious. Continue to learn, adapt, and grow. This journey, while rooted in ancient wisdom, thrives on contemporary discoveries.

**7. Looking Ahead**

As we near the end of this book, I want to leave you with a thought: the fasting journey, much like life, isn't about a destination—it's about the voyage. The learnings, the discoveries, the challenges, and the breakthroughs all amalgamate into an experience that's uniquely yours.

So, as you turn this page and perhaps close this book, know that the journey doesn't end here. It continues. In the choices you make, the foods you savor, the moments of stillness, and the bustling days of activity, the journey unfolds. Embrace it, cherish it, and celebrate every step.

Thank you for allowing me to be a part of your story. Here's to the lifelong journey ahead.

# Free eBook: Digital Detox to Unplug & Heal: Navigating a World Without Screens

Want a free eBook teaching you how to do a digital detox and heal your brain from device addiction?

Visit our website to grab a free copy today!

www.selfhelp.academy

Printed in Great Britain
by Amazon